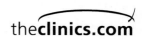

DENTAL CLINICS
OF NORTH AMERICA

Successful Esthetic and
Cosmetic Dentistry for the
Modern Dental Practice

GUEST EDITORS
John R. Calamia, DMD,
Mark S. Wolff, DDS, PhD, and
Richard J. Simonsen, DDS, MS

April 2007 • Volume 51 • Number 2

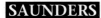

SAUNDERS

An Imprint of Elsevier, Inc.
PHILADELPHIA LONDON TORONTO MONTREAL SYDNEY TOKYO

W.B. SAUNDERS COMPANY
A Division of Elsevier Inc.

Elsevier Inc. • 1600 John F. Kennedy Boulevard • Suite 1800 • Philadelphia, Pennsylvania 19103-2899

http://www.dental.theclinics.com

DENTAL CLINICS OF NORTH AMERICA	**Volume 51, Number 2**
April 2007	**ISSN 0011-8532**
Editor: John Vassallo; j.vassallo@elsevier.com	**ISBN-13: 978-1-4160-4303-4**
	ISBN-10: 1-4160-4303-9

Reprints: For copies of 100 or more, of articles in this publication, please contact the Commercial Reprints Department, Elsevier Inc., 360 Park Avenue South, New York, New York, 10010-1710. Tel.: (212) 633-3813, Fax: (212) 462-1935, email: reprints@elsevier.com.

The ideas and opinions expressed in *The Dental Clinics of North America* do not necessarily reflect those of the Publisher. The Publisher does not assume any responsibility for any injury and/or damage to persons or property arising out of or related to any use of the material contained in this periodical. The reader is advised to check the appropriate medical literature and the product information currently provided by the manufacturer of each drug to be administered to verify the dosage, the method and duration of administration, or contraindications. It is the responsibility of the treating physician or other health care professional, relying on independent experience and knowledge of the patient, to determine drug dosages and the best treatment for the patient. Mention of any product in this issue should not be construed as endorsement by the contributors, editors, or the Publisher of the product or manufacturers' claims.

Dental Clinics of North America (ISSN 0011-8532) is published quarterly by Elsevier Inc., 360 Park Avenue South, New York, NY 10010-1710. Months of issue are January, April, July, and October. Business and Editorial Offices: 1600 John F. Kennedy Boulevard, Suite 1800, Philadelphia, PA 19103-2899. Customer Service Office: 6277 Sea Harbor Drive, Orlando, FL 32887-4800. Periodicals postage paid at New York, NY and additional mailing offices. Subscription prices are $171.00 per year (US individuals), $281.00 per year (US institutions), $83.00 per year (US students), $204.00 per year (Canadian individuals), $347.00 per year (Canadian institutions), $116.00 per year (Canadian students), $231.00 per year (international individuals), $347.00 per year (international institutions), and $116.00 per year (international students). International air speed delivery is included in all *Clinics* subscription prices. All prices are subject to change without notice. **POSTMASTER:** Send address changes to *Dental Clinics of North America*, Elsevier Periodicals Customer Service, 6277 Sea Harbor Drive, Orlando, FL 32887-4800. Customer Service: 1-800-654-2452 (US). From outside of the US, call 1-407-345-4000.

The *Dental Clinics of North America* is covered in *Index Medicus, Current Contents/Clinical Medicine, ISI/BIOMED* and *Clinahl.*

Printed in the United States of America.

GUEST EDITORS

JOHN R. CALAMIA, DMD, Professor; and Director of Esthetics, Department of Cariology and Comprehensive Care, New York University College of Dentistry, New York, New York

MARK S. WOLFF, DDS, PhD, New York University College of Dentistry, New York, New York

RICHARD J. SIMONSEN, DDS, MS, Dean, Midwestern University College of Dental Medicine, Glendale, Arizona

CONTRIBUTORS

ANNE E. BEALL, PhD, Beall Research & Training, Inc., Chicago, Illinois

RAYMOND L. BERTOLOTTI, DDS, PhD, Clinical Professor, University of California, San Francisco School of Dentistry, San Francisco, California

CHRISTINE S. CALAMIA, DDS, Department of Biomaterials and Biomemetics, New York University College of Dentistry, New York, NY

JOHN R. CALAMIA, DMD, Professor; and Director of Esthetics, Department of Cariology and Comprehensive Care, New York University College of Dentistry, New York, New York

RICARDO M. CARVALHO, DDS, PhD, Associate Professor, Department of Prosthodontics, Bauru School of Dentistry, University of São Paulo, Bauru, São Paulo, Brazil

SANG-CHOON CHO, DDS, Ashman Department of Periodontology and Implant Dentistry, New York University College of Dentistry, New York, New York

STEPHEN J. CHU, DMD, MSD, CDT, Director, Advanced CE Program in Aesthetic Dentistry; and Clinical Associate Professor, Department of Periodontics and Implant Dentistry, New York University College of Dentistry, New York, New York

ANTHONY J. CLASSI, DMD, Ashman Department of Periodontology and Implant Dentistry, New York University College of Dentistry, New York, New York

NELSON R.F.A. DA SILVA, DDS, MSc, PhD, Assistant Professor, Department of Prosthodontics, New York University College of Dentistry, New York, New York

NICHOLAS C. DAVIS, DDS, MAGD, Associate Professor, Loma Linda University, School of Dentistry, Loma Linda, California

BRIAN EHRLICH, DDS, Ashman Department of Periodontology and Implant Dentistry, New York University College of Dentistry, New York, New York

NICOLAS ELIAN, DDS, Ashman Department of Periodontology and Implant Dentistry, New York University College of Dentistry, New York, New York

STUART FROUM, DDS, Ashman Department of Periodontology and Implant Dentistry, New York University College of Dentistry, New York, New York

GALIP GÜREL, MSc, Nisantasi, Istanbul, Turkey

ZIAD N. JALBOUT, DDS, Ashman Department of Periodontology and Implant Dentistry, New York University College of Dentistry, New York, New York

STEVEN R. JEFFERIES, MS, DDS, The Donald and Cecelia Platnick Professor of Restorative Dentistry; and Director of Biomaterials Research Laboratory, Department of Restorative Dentistry; and Director of Clinical Research, Temple University School of Dentistry, Philadelphia, Pennsylvania

ANGELA R. KAMER, DDS, MS, PhD, Ashman Department of Periodontology and Implant Dentistry, New York University College of Dentistry, New York, New York

PATRICIA W. KIHN, DDS, MS, Director, Regulatory Clinical Support Activities, DENTSPLY International, Inc., York, Pennsylvania; Volunteer Faculty, Deans Faculty, Baltimore College of Dental Surgery, University of Maryland; Private Practice, Baltimore, Maryland

VINCENT G. KOKICH, DDS, MSD, Professor, Department of Orthodontics, University of Washington, Seattle, Washington

BRIAN P. LESAGE, DDS, Director, Beverly Hills Institute of Dental Esthetics; Director, UCLA Aesthetic Continuum; and Lecturer, Department of Restorative Dentistry, UCLA Dental School, California

KENNETH S. MAGID, DDS, Director of Pre Doctoral Laser Dentistry; and Associate Clinical Professor, International and Honors Esthetics, Department of Cariology and Comprehensive Care, New York University College of Dentistry, New York

THIAGO A. PEGORARO, DDS, Department of Prosthodontics, Bauru School of Dentistry, University of São Paulo, Bauru, São Paulo, Brazil

JORGE PERDIGÃO, DMD, MS, PhD, Associate Professor, Division of Operative Dentistry, Department of Restorative Sciences, University of Minnesota, Minneapolis, Minnesota

CHERYL L. SERIO, DDS, Assistant Professor, Department of Care Planning and Restorative Sciences, University of Mississippi School of Dentistry, Jackson, Mississippi

RICHARD J. SIMONSEN, DDS, MS, Dean, College of Dental Medicine, Midwestern University, Glendale, Arizona

FRANK M. SPEAR, DDS, MSD, Director, Seattle Institute for Advanced Dental Education, Seattle, Washington

HOWARD E. STRASSLER, DMD, Professor and Director of Operative Dentistry, Department of Endodontics, Prosthodontics and Operative Dentistry, University of Maryland Dental School, Baltimore, Maryland

ROBERT A. STRAUSS, DDS, MD, Director, Residency Training Program; and Professor of Surgery, Division of Oral and Maxillofacial Surgery, Department of Surgery, Virginia Commonwealth University Medical Center, Richmond, Virginia

DENNIS P. TARNOW, DDS, Ashman Department of Periodontology and Implant Dentistry, New York University College of Dentistry, New York, New York

CONTENTS

A smile has a tremendous impact on perceptions of one's attractiveness and one's personality. Previous psychological research
has shown that attractive people are perceived as more successful,
intelligent, and friendly. Research extends these findings by demonstrating that teeth alone can have an impact on overall attractiveness and perceptions of personality attributes. The results of
the study discussed in this article extend the attractiveness research
and demonstrate that one's smile is an important part of the physical attractiveness stereotype. One's smile clearly plays a significant role in the perception that others have of our appearance
and our personality.

Many scientific and artistic principles considered collectively are
useful in creating a beautiful smile. The evaluation and analysis
of the face, lips, gingival tissues and teeth are all considered in this
process. Recognizing the ideal as a goal provides a direction for diagnosis and treatment planning for smile rejuvenation. This article
focuses on the dental and dental-facial composition involved in
smile design. Basic facial esthetics are reviewed as a guideline for
facial analysis.

including modifications of metal surface and resin chemistry. Porcelain adhesion is reviewed, including little-known methods that use silane but no hydrofluoric acid etching. Clinical protocols for use of metal and porcelain adhesives are presented.

Dental cements are designed to retain restorations, appliances, and post and cores in a stable and, presumably, long-lasting position in the oral environment. Conventional glass ionomer and zinc phosphate cements are among the most popular materials for luting metallic restorations and posts, whereas resin-based cements are preferred for esthetic applications. Successful cementation of esthetic restorations is largely dependent on the appropriate treatment and silane application to the internal surface of the restoration. Clinicians are frequently advised to use three-step total-etch or two-step self-etch adhesive for luting purposes to avoid problems of incompatibility between adhesives and chemical- or dual-cure cements. A reliable cementation procedure can only be achieved if the operator is aware of the mechanisms involved and the material limitations.

The shade matching of a restoration is the critical final step in aesthetic restorative dentistry once morphology and occlusion are addressed. This article describes a seven-step approach to successful shade matching: patient and tooth evaluation, image capture and shade analysis, communication, interpretation, fabrication, verification, and placement of restoration. A step-by-step protocol to shade matching is comprehensively outlined through a case study using a combination of technology-based instrumentation, conventional techniques, and reference photography.

Today's dentist does not just repair teeth to make them better for chewing. Increasingly, his or her work involves esthetics. With patients demanding more attractive teeth, dentists now must become more familiar with the formerly independent disciplines of orthodontics, periodontics, restorative dentistry, and maxillofacial surgery. This article provides a systematic method of evaluating dentofacial esthetics in a logical, interdisciplinary manner. In today's interdisciplinary dental world, treatment planning must begin with well-defined esthetic objectives. By beginning with esthetics, and taking into consideration the impact on function, structure, and biology, the clinician will be able to use the various disciplines in dentistry to deliver the highest level of dental care to each patient.

The primary reasons for splinting and stabilizing teeth are to connect them for the purpose of replacing missing teeth or as an adjunct to periodontal therapy. Although the restorations must be planned to withstand the functional requirements of occlusion and mastication, esthetic considerations must also be taken into account. The challenge in creating an esthetic result with fiber-reinforced composite splints is that there is limited space in the connector region to create the three-dimensional effect required to give teeth the appearance of individuality. Careful planning in the diagnosis and treatment of the fiber splint is essential to allow for adequate tooth preparation to give the illusion of nonsplinted teeth. When missing teeth are replaced with a fiber-reinforced, direct, fixed partial denture, the pontic must be created to achieve an esthetically pleasing result.

In esthetic dentistry, expanding the evaluation beyond the teeth is necessary to achieve a truly desirable result. The lips, attached and unattached mucosa, free gingival margin, and osseous position and contours must be considered and changed if necessary. Although many treatment modalities are available to accomplish these modifications, the use of lasers of varying wavelengths provides advantages not possible by other means. Lasers are often thought of as generic instruments, but different laser wavelengths function differently, and each has its place in the esthetic continuum. Diode, neodymium:YAG, CO_2 and erbium lasers each have advantages that can be exploited to maximum effect and disadvantages that must be taken into consideration. A thorough understanding of their mechanism of action, their tissue effects, and laser safety is vital to obtaining excellent results.

To obtain optimal and predictable aesthetics, deficiencies caused by soft and particularly hard tissue loss can be managed by various methods, such as orthodontic tooth eruption, socket preservation, and guided bone regeneration. However, in complex cases, these methods are often insufficient. Here, the authors introduce advanced concepts in aesthetic implant dentistry, such as "Aesthetic Site Foundation", "Aesthetic Guided Bone Regeneration" and "Implant Rectangle" that will guide the clinician in the quest to optimal aesthetic outcomes.

FORTHCOMING ISSUES

RECENT ISSUES

ELSEVIER
SAUNDERS

Dent Clin N Am 51 (2007) xv–xvi

THE DENTAL
CLINICS
OF NORTH AMERICA

Preface

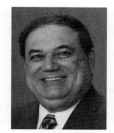 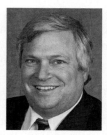 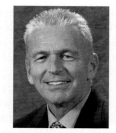

John R. Calamia, DMD   Mark S. Wolff, DDS, PhD   Richard J. Simonsen, DDS, MS

Guest Editors

I believe that few would argue against the premise that a basic body of knowledge of the aesthetic and cosmetic restoration of the human dentition is paramount to the successful modern-day practice of dentistry in North America. Evidence-based information is sought by the student of esthetic and cosmetic dentistry, whether they are generalists, specialists, seasoned practitioners, or recent graduates.

As the Senior Editor of this issue of *Dental Clinics of North America*, I have tried to select authors and topics that will provide foundational information in a clear and factual text. As you read through the table of contents, I hope that you recognize the care in the selection of topics, which should provide readers with a great outline of philosophy of practice, perception of the needs of our patients, and articles that provide in-depth methods and techniques that are the most sought after and delivered procedures in modern practice.

In the first article (an editorial), a sense of the ethical questions that should be asked in developing one's philosophy of treatment, consistent with the best interests of our patients, is presented. This editorial challenges us to do the right thing in providing these often elective procedures. In the second article, a snapshot of the perception of our prospective patients in North America and their feelings about the importance of an aesthetically pleasing smile is provided. Like the editorial, this is a unique article for *Dental Clinics of North America*. It presents a factual survey that helps us garner the perceived value of a smile by a true cross-section of the US population.

0011-8532/07/$ - see front matter. Published by Elsevier Inc.
doi:10.1016/j.cden.2007.03.009

dental.theclinics.com

The articles that follow provide current and cutting-edge information on the modalities of treatment, methods, and materials that allow us to provide quality, long-lasting aesthetic restorations for our patients. The most conservative (least invasive) treatments are discussed first, followed by treatments and methods that are necessary for the more difficult, complicated, and multidisciplinary cases.

I am confident that this issue not only will become a significant reference to all who wish to provide modern dental care but also will be an important resource for modern dental educators in developing a curriculum of knowledge needed by a new generation of dental students. In so doing, these students will, upon graduation, hit the ground running in their practice of the profession of dentistry.

I would like to express my sincere appreciation to the internationally respected professionals who have, without financial reward, given generously of their expertise and time despite their many commitments. They each have submitted excellent work for this color edition, and I want to thank them for their excellent cooperation with me and my co-editors, Dr. Mark Wolff and Dr. Richard Simonsen. Finally, I would like to thank my wife, Dr. Sonia Calamia, my daughter, Dr. Christine Calamia, and my son, current dental student and future dentist, Vincent J. Calamia, for their support in this endeavor.

John R. Calamia

John R. Calamia, DMD
Department of Cariology and Comprehensive Care
New York University College of Dentistry
345 East 24th Street, New York, NY 10010-4086, USA

E-mail address: jrc1@nyu.edu

Mark S. Wolff, DDS, PhD
New York University College of Dentistry
Room 1607 VAMC, MC 9480, 345 East 24th Street
New York, NY 10010-4086, USA

E-mail address: mark.wolff@nyu.edu

Richard J. Simonsen, DDS, MS
Midwestern University College of Dental Medicine
19555 North 59th Avenue, Glendale, AZ 85308, USA

E-mail address: rsimon@midwestern.edu

ELSEVIER
SAUNDERS

THE DENTAL
CLINICS
OF NORTH AMERICA

Dent Clin N Am 51 (2007) 281–287

Editorial

Commerce versus Care: Troubling Trends in the Ethics of Esthetic Dentistry

Where is the professional and public outrage at the troubling trends in the marketing and selling of "cosmetic" dentistry that besiege our profession today?

The code of primum non nocere—first and foremost do no harm—seems to have been cast aside in the headlong pursuit of outrageous overtreatment for financial gain by some. Fortunately, this trend is manifest by a small, although unfortunately highly visible, minority in the profession. Their actions, however, affect all in the dental profession, as the public begins to understand what is being sold to them in the name of "changing lives."

The American Dental Association's "Principles of Ethics and Code of Professional Conduct" states,

> The dental professional holds a special position of trust within society. As a consequence, society affords the profession certain privileges that are not available to members of the public-at-large. In return, the profession makes a commitment to society that its members will adhere to high ethical standards of conduct [1].

Thus, there is an implied contract between the dental profession and society. One would expect, therefore, outrage, or at least umbrage, to be shown by society (and from fellow members of the profession) if the implied contract is pushed to its limits, as I believe is happening today, with the balance between commerce versus care tilting toward commerce at the expense of care.

There are several ethical issues that should concern us all, such as

- the use of false or nonrecognized credentials promoted by nonaccredited institutions
- reliance on unproved science to promote treatments
- exaggeration of clinical skills and education
- unnecessary treatment and services
- lack of full informed consent
- harmful practices, such as the unnecessary removal of tooth structure and the replacement of highly clinically successful materials (such as gold) with inferior, untested restorative materials

doi:10.1016/j.cden.2007.03.002

- exposing patients to the unknown risks of overtreatment
- excessive fees
- failure to refer to specialists

When considering elective cosmetic enhancement, patient health always should come first in the mind of practitioners and always should trump patients' cosmetic desires, even at the expense of patient autonomy. Woe to clinicians who allow personal economic goals, masked beneath patients' naïvely expressed cosmetic desires, to lead to unnecessary or excessive treatment. We, as a profession, have an ethical duty to weigh the benefits and the risks of any procedure, and if the potential harm or risks outweigh the benefits, even patients' requests for treatment should be declined. That decision is the appropriate application of professional judgment by the dental profession, on which society relies, in the manner of the implied contract with the profession.

I am not an expert in ethics. I did not know as a college student that I one day would regret having focused so much on the sciences at the expense of the arts—in other words, I did not know what I did not know. Much to my later chagrin, I never took even as much as an introductory course in philosophy. So, my opinions come from inside. They are based on what my parents, and my school, Portsmouth Grammar School in Portsmouth, England, taught me about what is right and wrong. So, like my interest in grammar, where I do not really know all the rules but I certainly know what is right and wrong by how something sounds, so it is with ethics. I do not know all the rules. I have not read the writings of Aquinas or Aristotle, Descartes or Kant. I simply am relating how I believe ethics affects us as dentists in the practice of our profession based on my inner feelings of what is right and what is wrong. And where I see wrong, I believe it is my, and collectively our, duty to say something or become a part of the problem as enablers of unethical diagnosis and treatment.

The field of ethics involves concepts of right and wrong behavior. Generally, the field, as I understand it, is divided into three general subject areas: metaethics, normative ethics, and applied ethics. The areas that I focus on are the area of normative ethics and the subareas of duty theories and consequentialist theories (yes, I looked up the official terminology!) [2].

The seventeenth-century German philosopher, Samuel Pufendorf, classified dozens of duties under several headings. I confine this discussion to Pufendorf's descriptions of duties toward others and his rights theory [2]. Rights and duties are related inasmuch as the rights of one could be the duty of another. A "right" is a justified claim against someone else's behavior—for example, patients' right not to be harmed by dentists. Duties can be divided into absolute duties that are universally binding on people and conditional duties that stem from contracts between people (keeping promises). One can recognize in the absolute duties (avoiding wronging others, treating people as equals, and promoting the good of others) the basis for how most of us are raised by our parents, and I believe I can recognize in how these duties were impressed on me the reasons why I feel the way I do about the state of our profession when it comes to ethics, in particular our ethical understanding of cosmetic dentistry.

A more recent duty-based theory is proposed by the British philosopher, W.D. Ross, which emphasizes prima facie duties [2]. Ross's list of duties is as follows:

- fidelity: the duty to keep promises
- reparation: the duty to compensate others when we harm them
- gratitude: the duty to thank those who help us
- justice: the duty to recognize merit
- beneficence: the duty to improve the conditions of others
- self-improvement: the duty to improve our virtue and intelligence
- nonmaleficence: the duty to not injure others

Moral responsibility also can be determined by assessing the consequences of our actions (consequentialist theory). Accordingly, an action is morally right if the consequences of that action are more favorable than unfavorable [2].

Bader and Shugars [3] state,

> An implicit, if not explicit, assumption accompanying any treatment is that the benefits of the treatment will, or at least are likely to, outweigh any negative consequences of the treatment. . .in short, that treatment is better than no treatment.

Thus, if the potential harm from any treatment, in particular an elective intervention, exceeds the potential benefit, then it is unethical to carry out that particular treatment or enhancement. For example, placing 8 or 10 veneers for a patient who needs the esthetic enhancement of one tooth, thus starting the patient on a cycle of never-ending restorative treatment for many teeth from which the patient never can be extricated, properly can be termed, beneficence gone wild.

When I attended dental school (1967–1971), the prevailing doctrine of the times was a paternalistic, hippocratic approach to dentistry. We, as dentists, my teachers told me, know best and if patients do not like what we propose for treatment, they should be shown the door. Patients who are not good at following oral hygiene instructions are told they could not be treated until they shaped up. Patients even should be coerced into treatment (for their own good, of course) and patient autonomy was a weak principle in the dental educational system of the time. Dentists, or physicians, know best.

By the turn of the century, the pendulum thankfully had swung greatly from the paternalistic attitudes of decades past to increased patient autonomy and full informed consent for all treatment. Informed consent is the practice of informing a patient fully about all aspects of interventions relevant to patients' choice between authorizing or refusing a proposed course of therapy and enabling them to make a choice about an intervention.

Informed consent includes reinforcing the option of no treatment. It is dentists' responsibility to decline to carry out a treatment if it involves the unnecessary, or avoidable, destruction of healthy tooth structure.

Unfortunately, my view of some cases I see presented in the dental tabloids leads me to the conclusion that many offices where cosmetic dentistry procedures are marketed pay only lip service to accurate and full informed consent procedures, and this is true in particular for the no-treatment option. In some of the cases I have observed, it is hard for me to understand that patients could have been informed appropriately, or they surely would have chosen alternative, more conservative options, including possibly no treatment, rather than starting on a life cycle of restorative treatment [4]. This last option of no treatment is, of course, contrary to financial self-interests, although not of the ethical contractual bond, of dentists who are bent on increasing productivity.

Any elected treatment should be made only after full and complete informed consent, with all treatment options presented in an unbiased fashion. It seems as if some colleagues use claims of informed consent as a means to divert criticism. We must realize that informed consent is ignored, in many instances, by clinicians or patients. When I visit an expert, am I going to second-guess what I believe is the expert's opinion? In most cases, I am not. As patients, we all tend to go along with what health care practitioners expert advise.

Recent trends to promote office production, above any concerns for patients, are troubling. As Fuchs [5,6] notes in a recent editorial, originally published in the Missouri State Dental Journal, *Focus MDA*, and reprinted in the *ADA News*, "Could it be that over the last two decades dentists have drifted from being patient advocates to the current wildly popular 'practice advocates'?" We are inundated with articles and magazines on how to increase office income, and it is not hard to see that the best-attended courses, when it comes to continuing education, always seem to be the courses that promise greater income and how to get patients to say "yes" to financially rewarding treatment plans. That is truly sad in a profession, such as ours, that is based in service, in preventing and treating disease, and in restoring health.

Ozar and Sokol [7] proposed a hierarchy of values, which became an excellent tool for ranking professional values. Sometimes the choice is between the lesser of two evils when it comes to choosing between patient desires based on their knowledge level and the appropriate treatment from a clinician point of view. Ozar and Sokol's hierarchy lists the values as follows:

1. the patient's life and general health
2. the patient's oral health
3. the patient's autonomy
4. the dentist's preferred pattern of practice
5. esthetic values
6. efficiency in the use of resources

The rule of the hierarchy is that it is unethical to take any action that puts a lower item on the list ahead of a higher item on the list. In other words, as an example, a patient's oral health always trumps esthetic values. Similarly, a clinician is acting unethically if "he or she chose to provide treatment to a patient that enhanced the patient's oral health and yet put the patient's general health in jeopardy" [8].

If clinicians hang their hats exclusively on the duty of nonmaleficence, it follows that treatments of no effectiveness (as long as they do no obvious short-term harm and patients insist on getting the treatment) are acceptable. If, however, one holds to the duty of beneficence also, as we all should, then one must practice at a higher ethical standard than performing treatments that have no effect on patient health. How does one know, for example, that placing 8 or 10 veneers does no harm? What if the esthetic benefit is minimal or even nonexistent? Is there a benefit that outweighs the negative aspects of a young person having to live with the inevitable consequences of a foreign material (no matter how good it is) that is attempting to replace natural enamel? Worse is the fact that some clinicians use materials, such as pressed ceramics, that lead to preparations that necessarily must be cut into the dentin to allow for adequate thickness of the material. Thus, vast amounts of otherwise healthy tooth structure are sacrificed in the name of cosmetics—an enhancement that clearly violates Ozar and Sokol's hierarchy.

As I struggle with my own thoughts on the issues of the ethics of cosmetic dentistry, I think back to a text that I wrote in the mid-1970's, published in 1978 [9]. In that text were several chapters on what today would be called cosmetic dentistry, inspired by what the new bonded resin materials could accomplish, for example, for patients who had a fractured central incisor, compared with the aggressive treatments indicated at the time as the standard of care. I have not checked, but I doubt that I used the word "cosmetic" in the book. That is because I never believed these treatments cosmetic, per se. In my mind, almost every clinical procedure we, as dentists, carry out has an esthetic component. What caught my attention were the minimally invasive options then possible that were of great benefit to patients in terms of the conservation of tooth structure with the use of resin composites and the acid-etch technique. Instead of a full crown on a central incisor, we simply could apply a resin composite and end up with an esthetic result that was in most cases indistinguishable from a crown. Of course, in those days, the color stability of the resins meant that the restorations had to be resurfaced or replaced in a short period of time. That is not true today with advances in application methods and with the excellent color stability of the modern resin materials.

In the early 1980s, John Calamia and I published the first information (in the form of an oral presentation and an abstract in the *Journal of Dental Research*) relating to the potential for etching porcelain for "anterior veneers and other intraoral uses" [10]. This was followed by Calamia's [11] landmark article on a clinical case. Again, at the time, my ideas were connected to the saving of tooth structure with these advances, not as much to the "cosmetic" benefits, as these benefits could be obtained in other ways using the esthetic techniques of the time, albeit sometimes with more aggressive tooth preparation. The idea for etching porcelain came from thinking about how we could improve the color-unstable resin composite veneers that were state of the art at that time. Using porcelain was an obvious benefit, but no one had thought of a way to accomplish that task. When thoughts of how to improve resin composite veneers were put together with the observation that dental laboratories routinely removed porcelain from discarded bridges to reclaim the gold with a liquid, the acid etching of porcelain for retention as a veneer became a reality. Calamia's first clinical case of etched porcelain veneers was done without removal of tooth structure, although the standard of care today reflects the minimally invasive preparation within enamel that has become routine.

Perhaps this conservative, minimally invasive philosophy that I have is responsible for the visceral repulsion I feel from some of the enhancement cases (I would not call them treatment, as this suggests a health benefit) I see published in the tabloid press. This leads to the crux of the ethical argument today over cosmetic dentistry. Although I believe that most dentists who concentrate on cosmetic enhancements are ethical and honest in their approach, the few who push the envelope of ethical responsibility and overtreat patients for financial gain are responsible for creating an environment where the commerce of dentistry is put first and patient care second. Spear wrote an excellent commentary on this problem in a recent issue of the *Journal of the American Dental Association*, ending with, "Providing occlusal therapy is a health care service first, a business and financial resource second" [12].

I began this editorial with the question, "Where is the outrage?" Already, that question suggests a certain bias in the topic and the situation we are facing in dentistry today. I have no argument with general practitioners who wish to become more adept at esthetic procedures and who focus interest in taking courses designed to improve clinical skills in esthetic, or cosmetic, dentistry. Where I have issue is with those who go to a couple of weekend courses at an "institute" and then advertise that they are expert in full mouth reconstruction, a level of skill that prosthodontic colleagues study full time for 3 or 4 years in graduate school to attain. The most dangerous among us are those who jump on the cosmetic bandwagon and who do not know what they do not know. Training in a formal, accredited residency program should be required of those who choose to market cosmetic dentistry aggressively, and full mouth reconstruction should be left to prosthodontic colleagues.

So, where is the outrage at what is going on in our profession? The problem is not that cosmetic procedures should not be done; minimally invasive esthetic correction can be a wonderful service when diagnosed ethically and presented to patients. The problem is that cosmetic dentistry should not be aggressively overpromoted and sold to the public, as increasingly is happening today. Dentists need to get back to being patient advocates. In doing so, the practice income will take care of itself.

The ethics of esthetic dentistry needs to get back on course before outrage breaks loose and Big Brother decides to take care of us, because we cannot take care of the dental professional ethics and professional conduct ourselves. That will be a sad day for the profession's autonomy. As one of the founders of the Mayo Clinic, William Mayo, once put it, "The best interest of the patient, is the only interest to be considered." Where treatment planning in esthetic dentistry is concerned, that should be the profession's mantra.

Richard J. Simonsen, DDS, MS
Dean, College of Dental Medicine
Midwestern University
19555 North 59th Avenue
Glendale, AZ 85308, USA

E-mail address: rsimon@midwestern.edu

References

[1] Principles of ethics and code of professional conduct. American Dental Association. Available at: http://www.ada.org/prof/prac/law/code/index.asp. Accessed February 16, 2007.
[2] The internal encyclopedia of philosophy. Available at: http://www.iep.utm.edu/e/ethics.htm. Accessed February 16, 2007.
[3] Bader JD, Shugars DA. Variation, treatment outcomes and practice guidelines in dental practice. J Dent Educ 1995;59(1):61–5.
[4] Simonsen RJ. New materials on the horizon. J Am Dent Assoc 1991;122:25–31.
[5] Fuchs DJ. Ethical equation: why aren't we No. 1? ADA News 2006;38:4–5.
[6] Christensen GJ. I have had enough! DentalTown magazine 2003;4(9):10–2.
[7] Ozar DT, Sokol DJ. Dental ethics at chairside: professional principles and practical applications. Georgetown University Press, 2nd edition. Washington, DC, 1994.
[8] Jenson L. My way or the highway: do dental patients really have autonomy? Issues in dental ethics. J Am Coll Dent 2003;70(1):26–30.
[9] Simonsen RJ. Clinical applications of the acid etch technique. Chicago: Quintessence Publishing Co.; 1978.
[10] Simonsen RJ, Calamia JR. Tensile bond strengths of etched porcelain. J Dent Res 1983;62: 297 [abstract no. 1154].
[11] Calamia JR. Etched porcelain facial veneers: a new treatment modality based on scientific and clinical evidence. NY J Dent 1983;53(6):255–9.
[12] Spear FM. The business of occlusion. J Am Dent Assoc 2006;137:666–7.

THE DENTAL
CLINICS
OF NORTH AMERICA

Dent Clin N Am 51 (2007) 289–297

Can a New Smile Make You Look More Intelligent and Successful?

Anne E. Beall, PhD

Beall Research & Training, Inc., 203 N. Wabash, Suite 1308, Chicago, IL 60601, USA

One of the intriguing findings in psychological research is the existence of a physical attractiveness stereotype. Researchers have found that people believe that beautiful individuals are happier, sexually warmer, more outgoing, more intelligent, and more successful than their less attractive counterparts [1–3]. Research on cosmetic surgery has shown this effect in its strongest form. One study used photographs of women before and after cosmetic surgery and found that the pictured women were perceived as more physically attractive, kinder, more sensitive, sexually warmer, more responsive, and more likable after surgery than before it [4].

Although the physical attractiveness stereotype has been demonstrated with overall attractiveness, the role teeth play in perceptions of overall attractiveness has never been established. It has never been ascertained whether appealing teeth alone can influence perceptions of one's personality. This research study investigates these two questions. (The American Academy of Cosmetic Dentistry commissioned Beall Research & Training, Inc. to conduct this study to ascertain what impact attractive teeth have on perceptions of an individual's appearance and personality attributes.)

Research design

This research used a between-subject's design in which one half of respondents viewed one set of pictures (Set A) and the other half viewed another set of pictures (Set B) (Table 1). Sets A and B comprised pictures of individuals in which one half of all photos were of a person with a "before" smile and the other half were with people with a smile "after" cosmetic dentistry. No respondent ever saw the same person with a "before" and "after" smile; however, all respondents viewed the same set of eight individuals.

E-mail address: beallrt@sbcglobal.net

Table 1
Picture sets used in study

Picture set A	Picture set B	Change
Female pictures		
Maribel (*before smile*)	Maribel (*after smile*)	Major
Stephanie (*after smile*)	Stephanie (*before smile*)	Major
Kathy (*after smile*)	Kathy (*before smile*)	Moderate
Shelley (*before smile*)	Shelley (*after smile*)	Minor
Male pictures		
Jim (*before smile*)	Jim (*after smile*)	Major
Mike (*after smile*)	Mike (*before smile*)	Major
Milt (*before smile*)	Milt (*after smile*)	Moderate
Bob (*after smile*)	Bob (*before smile*)	Minor

Fig. 1 contains one picture set that was shown. (To see all pictures used in this study, please visit www.aacd.com.) One half of the pictures were of men and the other half were of women. Each picture was classified in terms of the degree of change between the "before" and "after" smile. Four of the photos involved patients who underwent major changes, two underwent moderate changes, and two showed minor changes. After seeing each picture, respondents rated each person on the following attributes:

- Attractive
- Intelligent
- Happy
- Successful in their career
- Friendly
- Interesting
- Kind
- Wealthy
- Popular with the opposite sex
- Sensitive to other people

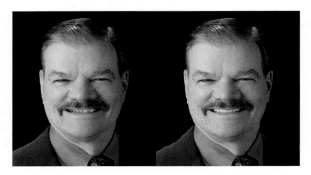

Fig. 1. Picture example (Bob). One half of respondents saw the picture on the left and the other half of respondents saw the picture on the right. (*Courtesy of* American Academy of Cosmetic Dentistry, Madison, WI; with permission.)

Respondents used a 1 to 10 scale, in which "1" represented "not at all" and "10" represented "extremely." A rating of "10" on the first attribute would indicate that the respondent thought the pictured person was "extremely attractive." Photos and ratings were randomized to eliminate order effects. All photos were randomized for each respondent along with the order of the rated attributes.

We conducted this study with a national sample of the US population. Completion quotas were set for age groups, income groups, geographic region and gender to represent the US population. The percentage of respondents in each quota category is shown at the end of this document along with the percentage of individuals for that category of the US population.

We conducted this study over the Internet. Five hundred twenty-eight respondents completed the survey. This sample size yields a confidence interval of ±4%, which means that the true answer for the US population is ±4%.

Statistical analyses

All statistical analyses were conducted on the mean ratings, which are shown in Tables 2 and 3. We conducted a paired T-test, which is a statistical test of significance that is designed to establish if a difference exists between sample means. In this research, that result is the difference between the mean rating of people with "before" smiles and the mean rating of people with "after" smiles. Statistically speaking, the T-test is the ratio of the variance that occurs between the sample means to the variance occurring within the sample groups. A large T-value occurs when the variance between groups is larger than the variance within groups. Large T-values indicate a significant difference between the sample means.

Table 2
T-statistics for each attribute

Attribute	Rating of "before" smile[a]	Rating of "after" smile[a]	T-statistic	Significance
Attractive	4.63	5.89	25.81	<.0001
Intelligent	5.85	6.51	16.11	<.0001
Happy	6.22	6.82	13.59	<.0001
Successful in their career	5.76	6.69	20.87	<.0001
Friendly	6.26	6.75	11.94	<.0001
Interesting	5.43	6.12	16.34	<.0001
Kind	5.98	6.40	10.37	<.0001
Wealthy	4.93	5.89	20.27	<.0001
Popular with the opposite sex	5.00	6.18	23.61	<.0001
Sensitive to other people	5.65	6.10	10.97	<.0001

[a] Composite mean.

Table 3
T-statistics arrayed by strongest effects

Attribute	Rating of "before" smile[a]	Rating of "after" smile[a]	T-statistic	Significance
Attractive	4.63	5.89	25.81	<.0001
Popular with the opposite sex	5.00	6.18	23.61	<.0001
Successful in their career	5.76	6.69	20.87	<.0001
Wealthy	4.93	5.89	20.27	<.0001
Interesting	5.43	6.12	16.34	<.0001
Intelligent	5.85	6.51	16.11	<.0001
Happy	6.22	6.82	13.59	<.0001
Friendly	6.26	6.75	11.94	<.0001
Sensitive to other people	5.65	6.10	10.97	<.0001
Kind	5.98	6.40	10.37	<.0001

[a] Composite mean.

We conducted a paired T-test on each attribute individually. We looked at the mean rating for the "before" smile and the "after" smile and determined if this difference was statistically significant. Because each respondent rated eight different pictures, we created a composite mean of their ratings for the "before" smile pictures and the "after" smile pictures. The T-test was conducted on these composite means.

Major results

The results of the T-tests are shown in Table 2. This statistical analysis demonstrated that there is a major effect of a smile on perceptions of all major attributes. In each case, people are viewed as more attractive, intelligent, happy, successful in their career, friendly, interesting, kind, wealthy, and popular with the opposite sex with smiles that have been altered by cosmetic dentistry versus their original smiles. Table 2 contains the T-statistic for each attribute.

These attributes also can be arrayed in terms of the strongest effects—the largest T-statistics. Table 3 contains the information from Table 2 as ranked by the size of the T-statistic. The attributes of being attractive, popular with the opposite sex, successful in their career, and wealthy had the largest T-statistics. These attributes had a higher mean for the "after" smile, however, and were all statistically significantly different.

Type of change

We also looked at the amount of change between the "before" and "after" smile and classified the changes as major, moderate, and minor. These classifications were observational and were not validated in any way. They were included because we wanted to show a range of changes because it is likely that cosmetic dentistry is done for various smiles in actual practice. The data in Table 4 show the mean ratings for the "before" and "after" smile for each type of change.

As the data show, the major changes showed the largest mean differences between the "before" and "after" smiles. These differences ranged from 0.6 to 1.9. Moderate changes showed a mean difference that ranged from 0.3 to 0.8. Not surprisingly, minor changes showed the smallest mean differences, which ranged from 0.2 to 0.6 (see Table 4).

Table 4
Ratings for major, moderate, and minor changes in smile

Attributes	"Before smile" mean (n = 264)	"After smile" mean (n = 264)	Difference
Major changes			
Attractive	4.5	6.4	1.9
Intelligent	5.7	6.7	1.0
Happy	6.2	7.0	0.8
Successful in their career	5.5	6.8	1.3
Friendly	6.3	7.0	0.7
Interesting	5.4	6.5	1.1
Kind	6.0	6.6	0.6
Wealthy	4.6	6.0	1.4
Popular with the opposite sex	5.0	6.7	1.7
Sensitive to other people	5.7	6.3	0.6
Moderate changes			
Attractive	4.6	5.3	0.7
Intelligent	5.9	6.3	0.4
Happy	6.2	6.7	0.5
Successful in their career	5.7	6.4	0.7
Friendly	6.4	6.8	0.4
Interesting	5.4	5.9	0.5
Kind	6.1	6.4	0.3
Wealthy	4.8	5.4	0.6
Popular with the opposite sex	4.9	5.7	0.8
Sensitive to other people	5.8	6.1	0.3
Minor changes			
Attractive	4.8	5.4	0.6
Intelligent	6.1	6.4	0.3
Happy	6.2	6.4	0.2
Successful in their career	6.4	6.9	0.5
Friendly	6.1	6.3	0.2
Interesting	5.5	5.7	0.2
Kind	5.8	6.0	0.2
Wealthy	5.7	6.2	0.5
Popular with the opposite sex	5.1	5.6	0.5
Sensitive to other people	5.4	5.7	0.3

In general, the largest differences between the "before" and "after" smile for each type of change occurred for the attributes of being attractive, successful in their career, wealthy, and popular with the opposite sex.

Gender of pictured person

Table 5 shows the ratings for "before" and "after" smile pictures of men and women. The difference in ratings for male pictures ranged from 0.4 to 1.2, with the largest differences occurring for attributes of being attractive, popular with the opposite sex, and successful in their career. For women, the difference ranged from 0.4 to 1.3, with the largest differences occurring for attributes of being attractive, popular with the opposite sex, and wealthy. These tables clearly demonstrate that the effect of cosmetic dentistry is seen with male and female pictures.

Demographics

This study imposed strict quotas for geographic region, age, household income, and gender. Table 6 shows the percentage of respondents in each category. The final respondents are representative of the US population in terms of region, age, income, and gender.

Table 5
Ratings for male and female pictures

Attributes	"Before smile" mean (n = 264)	"After smile" mean (n = 264)	Difference
Male pictures			
Attractive	4.7	5.9	1.2
Intelligent	5.9	6.5	0.6
Happy	6.2	6.8	0.6
Successful in their career	5.7	6.7	1.0
Friendly	6.2	6.7	0.5
Interesting	5.5	6.2	0.7
Kind	6.0	6.4	0.4
Wealthy	5.1	6.0	0.9
Popular with the opposite sex	5.1	6.2	1.1
Sensitive to other people	5.7	6.1	0.4
Female pictures			
Attractive	4.5	5.8	1.3
Intelligent	5.8	6.6	0.8
Happy	6.3	6.9	0.6
Successful in their career	5.8	6.7	0.9
Friendly	6.3	6.8	0.5
Interesting	5.4	6.1	0.7
Kind	6.0	6.4	0.4
Wealthy	4.8	5.8	1.0
Popular with the opposite sex	4.9	6.1	1.2
Sensitive to other people	5.6	6.1	0.5

Table 6
Demographics of study

N = 528	Sample percentage (%)	US population percentage (%)
Region		
Northeast	18	19
Midwest	22	22
South	37	36
West	23	23
Age		
18–24 years old	12	12
25–34 years old	18	18
35–44 years old	21	20
45–54 years old	20	19
55–64 years old	15	14
65 or older	16	16
Household income		
<$20,000 per year	23	22
$20,000–$49,999 per year	33	33
$50,000–$74,999 per year	18	18
$75,000–$99,999 per year	11	11
≥$100,000 per year	16	16
Gender		
Male	52	49
Female	49	51

Data from US Census Bureau: Population Estimates GCT-T1: 2005 Population Estimates; US Census Bureau/2004 American Community Survey; US Census: Annual Demographic Survey HINC-01: Selected Characteristics of Households by Total Money Income 2004; US Census Bureau/2004 American Community Survey. Available at: http://www.factfinder.census.gov.

Discussion

The data from this study clearly demonstrate that a smile has a tremendous impact on perceptions of one's attractiveness and one's personality. Previous psychological research has shown that attractive people are perceived as more successful, intelligent, and friendly. This research extends these findings by demonstrating that the teeth alone can have an impact on overall attractiveness and perceptions of personality attributes.

The strongest effect of a smile is for attractiveness and being popular with the opposite sex. Popularity with the other gender is likely a proxy measure of attractiveness. Similarly strong effects occur for perceptions of being successful in one's career and being wealthy. These measures are somewhat similar, and it is possible that people believe that when one is successful, one tends to be wealthy. Other strong effects occur for being interesting, intelligent, happy, friendly, sensitive to others, and kind. For each of these attributes, people with smiles altered by cosmetic dentistry were regarded as having more of the attribute—as being more interesting, intelligent, and happy—than people with their original smiles.

These effects were observed for male and female pictures. Not surprisingly, the impact of a smile was less pronounced for minor changes in the

"before" and "after" smile than for moderate and major changes. It is noticeable, however, that the mean rating was higher for all attributes on the
"after" smile than for the "before" smile, even for minor changes.

So how true are these stereotypes? Research has demonstrated that attractive people are somewhat more relaxed and outgoing and have more social finesse than less attractive individuals [2,5]. In one research study, men
talked with several women for 5 minutes over the phone and then rated each
woman. The women who were most attractive were rated as more socially
skillful and likable.

What about being successful and wealthy? In a national study of Canadians, researchers rated individuals on a 1 to 5 attractiveness scale. They
found that for each additional scale of attractiveness, people earned an
additional $1988 annually [6]. This finding has been replicated in the United
States with MBA students [7]. Researchers demonstrated that for each additional scale unit of attractiveness, the men earned an additional $2600
per month and the women earned an additional $2150. Both of these studies
were conducted in the 1990s, so one can imagine what the dollar amounts
would be now.

It is possible that there is a self-fulfilling prophecy at work. Because people expect attractive individuals to be more intelligent, successful, and likable, they treat them in ways that engender these behaviors. Expectations
for others have been shown to have a tremendous impact on how we treat
people and how they behave in return, which leads to a self-fulfilling prophecy [8]. The more the behaviors are confirmed, the more we tend to believe in
our expectations. It is also possible that because people treat attractive
people in certain ways, attractive individuals begin to develop more social
self-confidence and greater self-esteem than their unattractive counterparts.

The results of this study extend the attractiveness research and demonstrate that one's smile is an important part of the physical attractiveness stereotype. One's smile clearly plays a significant role in the perception that
others have of our appearance and our personality.

References

[1] Eagly AH, Ashmore RD, Makhijani MG, et al. What is beautiful is good, but...: a meta-
    analytic review of the research on the physical attractiveness stereotype. Psychol Bull 1991;
    110:109–28.
[2] Feingold A. Good looking people are not what we think. Psychol Bull 1992;111:304–41.
[3] Jackson LA, Hunter JE, Hodge CN. Physical attractiveness and intellectual competence:
    a meta-analytic review. Soc Psychol Q 1995;58(2):108–22.
[4] Kalick SM. Plastic Surgery, physical appearance and person perception [Unpublished doc-
    toral dissertation]. Harvard University; 1977. [Cited by E. Berscheid in: An Overview of the
    psychological effects of physical attractiveness and some comments upon the psychological
    effects of knowledge of the effects of physical attractiveness. In: Lucker W, Ribbens K, &
    McNamera JA, Editors. Logical aspects of facial form. Ann Arbor: University of Michigan
    Press, 1981].

[5] Langlois JH, Kalakanis L, Rubenstein AJ, et al. Maxims or myths of beauty? A meta-analytic and theoretical review. Psychol Bull 2000;126:390–423.

[6] Roszell P, Kennedy D, Grabb E. Physical attractiveness and income attainment among Canadians. Journal of Psychology 1990;123:547–59.

[7] Frieze IH, Olson JE, Russell J. Attractiveness and income for men and women in management. J Appl Soc Psychol 1991;21:1039–57.

[8] Olson JM, Roese NJ, Zanna MP, Higgens ET. Expectancies. In: Kruglanski AW, editor. Social psychology: handbook of basic principles. New York: Guilford Press; 1996. p. 211–38.

THE DENTAL
CLINICS
OF NORTH AMERICA

Dent Clin N Am 51 (2007) 299–318

Smile Design

Nicholas C. Davis, DDS, MAGD*

*Loma Linda University, School of Dentistry, 11092 Anderson Street,
Loma Linda, CA 92354, USA*

Smile design refers to the many scientific and artistic principles that considered collectively can create a beautiful smile. These principles are established through data collected from patients, diagnostic models, dental research, scientific measurements, and basic artistic concepts of beauty. From the patient's perspective, beauty measures that individual's perception of beauty as noted in the saying: "Beauty is in the eye of the beholder." That perception of beauty may also be influenced by cultural, ethnic, or racial concepts of beauty and may vary from the standards established in the North American dental community.

When planning treatment for esthetic cases, smile design cannot be isolated from a comprehensive approach to patient care. Achieving a successful, healthy, and functional result requires an understanding of the interrelationship among all the supporting oral structures, including the muscles, bones, joints, gingival tissues, and occlusion. Gaining this understanding requires collecting all the data necessary to properly evaluate all the structures of the oral complex.

A comprehensive dental examination should include dental radiographs, mounted diagnostic models, photographic records, and a thorough clinical examination and patient interview. The clinical examination should include a smile analysis and the evaluation of the teeth, temporomandibular joints, occlusion, existing restorations, periodontal tissues, and other soft tissues of the oral cavity.

In addition to the esthetics, the function component of the anterior teeth must be considered in treatment planning. Anterior guidance in harmony with healthy joint positions is key in establishing a stable occlusal scheme. The strategic players in anterior guidance are the maxillary cuspids. A cuspid-protected occlusion helps improve the longevity of the occlusion,

* 1194 Morningside Drive, Laguna Beach, CA 92651.
E-mail address: info@smilesbydavis.com

anterior teeth, and aesthetic restorations. It also protects the periodontium by directing the occlusal forces along the long axis of the teeth. Guiding the function to eliminate lateral and occlusal interferences helps prevent fremetus and potential joint issues resulting from traumatic occlusion.

The principles of smile design require an integration of esthetic concepts that harmonize facial esthetics with the dental facial composition and the dental composition. The dental facial composition includes the lips and the smile as they relate to the face. The dental composition relates more specifically to the size, shape, and positions of the teeth and their relationship to the alveolar bone and gingival tissues. Therefore, smile design includes an evaluation and analysis of both the hard and soft tissues of the face and smile (Appendix 1).

This article focuses on the dental and dental–facial composition involved in smile design. Only basic facial esthetics are reviewed as a guideline for facial analysis. Analyzing, evaluating, and treating patients for the purpose of smile design often involve a multidiscipline approach to treatment. Specialty treatment for achieving an ideal smile can include orthodontics; orthognathic surgery; periodontal therapy, including soft tissue repositioning and bone recontouring; cosmetic dentistry; and plastic surgery. This esthetic approach to patient care produces the best dental and dental–facial beauty.

Facial beauty is based on standard esthetic principles that involve the proper alignment, symmetry, and proportions of the face. The basic shape of the face is derived from the scaffolding matrix comprised of the facial bones that form the skull and jaw as well as of the cartilage and soft tissues that overlay this framework.

Facial features in smile design include facial height, facial shape, facial profile, gender, and age. In classical terms, the face height is divided into three equal thirds: from forehead to brow line, from brow line to the base of the nose, and from the base of the nose to the base of the chin. The width of the face is typically the width of five "eyes" (Fig. 1) [1]. As viewed from the frontal position, the four basic facial shapes recognized in the Trubyte denture tooth mold selection guide are square, tapering, square tapering, and ovoid. Lateral facial profiles can be straight, convex, or concave. A cephalometric analysis of the head in frontal and lateral views is useful in determining bony relationships of the face and the mandible, and their relationship to the teeth in the alveolar bone. The facial features related to gender and age involve the soft tissues and include the texture, complexion, and tissue integrity of the epithelial tissues.

Facial features that have a particularly important impact on the dental–facial composition are those that relate the interpupillary plane with the commisure line and the occlusal plane [2]. The interpupillary line should be parallel with the horizon line and perpendicular to the midline of the face. In addition, the interpupillary line should be parallel with the commisure line and occlusal plane [3].

Lip analysis is another important soft tissue feature helpful in evaluating the dental–facial composition and establishing a smile design. The lips play

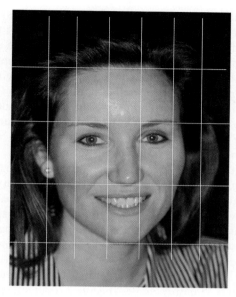

Fig. 1. Classical face proportions. (*Courtesy of* Nicholas C. Davis, DDS, MAGD, Loma Linda, CA.)

an important role in that they create the boundaries of the smile design's influence. Understanding lip morphology and lip mobility can often be helpful in meeting patients' expectations and determining the criteria for success.

Genetic traits; the position of the teeth, alveolar bone, and jaws; and their relationships influence the shape of the lips. The upper lip is somewhat more arched and wider than the lower lip. Because the maxillary arch with the teeth overlaps the mandibular arch, the upper lip is the longer of the two. The lower lip, therefore, is recessed beneath the upper lip approximately 30° in relation to the upper lip when the arches are properly aligned [4].

There are three aspects of the lip morphology that should be considered: width, fullness, and symmetry. Wide lips make for a wide smile. In general terms, a smile that is at least half the width of the face, at that level of the face, is considered esthetic. The fullness and symmetry of the upper and lower lips should also be documented. The fullness of the lip, or lip volume, can be categorized as full, average, or thin. Lip symmetry involves the mirror image appearance of each lip when smiling.

The upper and lower lips should be analyzed separately and independently of one another. Independent evaluation of the upper and lower lip is essential when analyzing both symmetry and fullness. The question should be asked: "Are the upper and lower lips symmetric on both sides of the midline and do they have the same degree of fullness?" In Fig. 2A, the upper and lower lips are symmetric but they differ in fullness. In Fig. 2B the upper lip is asymmetric and the lower lip is symmetric and the fullness is similar. Recognizing the etiology of lip asymmetries is helpful in determining if there is a dental solution for improvement or if plastic surgery is necessary. Some-times both are necessary to provide the results desired by the patient.

The position of the lips in the rest position should be evaluated for lip contact as well as for the range of lip mobility when smiling. These two determinants establish how much tooth structure and gingival tissue are revealed when comparing the repose and full smile positions. Evaluating this dental–facial feature can be helpful in analyzing and determining treat-ment modalities necessary to improve the smile. Lip evaluation is also useful when considering the patient's expectation and, more importantly, for revealing tooth and tissue asymmetries or defects.

When smiling, the inferior border of the upper lip as it relates to the teeth and gingival tissues is called the lip line. An average lip line exposes the max-illary teeth and only the interdental papillae. A high lip line exposes the teeth in full display as well as gingival tissues above the gingival margins. A low lip line displays no gingival tissues when smiling. In most cases, the lip line is acceptable if it is within a range of 2 mm apical to the height of the gingiva on the maxillary centrals [5].

In cases where there is a high lip line and an excessive gingival display exists, an unwanted "gummy smile" becomes evident. Several corrective options are available, depending on conditions and patient limitations. With cephalometric analysis, vertical maxillary excess can be determined. Orthodontics and orthognathic surgery to impact the maxilla are ideal when these conditions are confirmed as skeletal displasias in nature.

In other cases where apparent diminished tooth size in combination with a high lip line creates a gummy smile, corrective periodontal procedures are

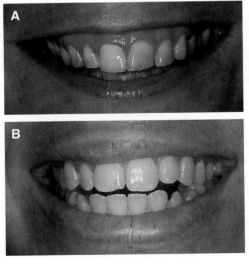

Fig. 2. (*A*) The upper and lower lips are symmetric but they differ in fullness. (*B*) The upper lip is asymmetric. (*Courtesy of* Nicholas C. Davis, DDS, MAGD, Loma Linda, CA.)

an option [6]. This involves cases where altered passive eruption makes a normal-sized tooth appear small. Altered passive eruption occurs when the pellicle does not completely recede to the cementoenamel junction [6]. As a result, the tooth appears short because the gingival portion of the enamel, which is usually exposed, remains covered with gingival tissues.

Cosmetic crown lengthening to expose the covered enamel can improve normal tooth height and tooth proportions. This can produce a more pleasing emergence profile of the tooth. These procedures can also be helpful in creating symmetry, positive radicular architecture, and proper zenith points of the gingival margins. Many times when exostosies exists, recontouring the alveolar bone is also necessary to recreate and define normal architecture and prevent a ledging appearance of the gingival tissues.

The frenum attachment can also affect the upper-lip shape and the amount of tooth exposure. In such cases, especially where the attachment is broad, a frenectomy that is dissected out from origin to insertion, removing the elastic fibers, can also free up the lip for normal lip movement. This can also be useful when a redundant flap of tissue, termed by this author as a "lip curtain" (Fig. 3), is visible hanging beneath the upper lip when smiling. These procedures, used in combination with cosmetic dental procedures, can reduce gummy smiles and produce a more esthetic smile (Fig. 4).

The incisal display refers to the amount of visible tooth displayed when the lips and lower jaw are in the rest position. The average incisal display of the maxillary centrals for males is 1.91 mm and the average for females is 3.40 mm [2]. With age, the amount of incisal display of the maxillary centrals diminishes and the amount of incisal display of the mandibular centrals increases [7]. Therefore, the amount of incisal display is an important factor in a youthful smile.

The inferior border of the upper lip and the superior border of the lower lip form an outline of the space that is revealed when smiling. The curvature of the lips as well as the prevalence of the shapes formed by the lips has been noted in texts [2]. The space that includes the teeth and tissues is called the smile zone [8]. There are six basic smile-zone shapes: straight, curved,

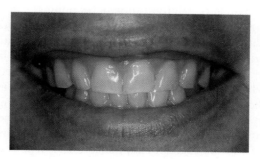

Fig. 3. A broad attachment of frenum creates second band of tissue, a "lip curtain," below the lip. (*Courtesy of* Nicholas C. Davis, DDS, MAGD, Loma Linda, CA.)

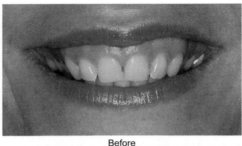

Before

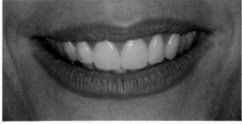

After

Fig. 4. Before (*top*) and after (*bottom*) crown lengthening, frenectomy and application of 10 maxillary porcelain veneers. (*Courtesy of* Nicholas C. Davis, DDS, MAGD, Loma Linda, CA.)

elliptical, bow-shaped, rectangular, and inverted (Fig. 5). The first three shapes are the most common. Identifying these shapes is helpful in analyzing the smile.

A feature of smile design that is often overlooked yet very significant is the health, symmetry, and architecture of the gingival tissues. These tissues frame the teeth and add to the symmetry of the smile. The health and subsequent color and texture of these gingival tissues are paramount for long-term success and the esthetic value of the treatment.

Healthy gingival tissues are pale pink and can vary in degree of vascularity, epithelial kertinization, and pigmentation, and in the thickness of the epithelium. The papillary contour should be pointed and should fill the interdental spaces to the contact point. An unfilled interdental space creates an unwanted black interdental triangle in the gingival embrasure and makes a smile less attractive (Fig. 6). Managing the soft tissues in this area improves the smile when these tissues are revealed. The architecture has a positive radicular shape forming a scalloped appearance that is symmetric on both sides of the midline. The marginal contour of the gingival should be sloped coronally to end in a thin edge. The texture of the tissues should be stippled (orange-peel–like appearance) in most cases. The stippling may be fine or coarse and the degree of stippling varies. In younger females, the tissue is more finely textured and has a finer stippling when compared with that of males. The tissue should be firm in consistency and the attached part

STRAIGHT   CURVED   ELLIPSE

BOW   RECTANGULAR   INVERTED

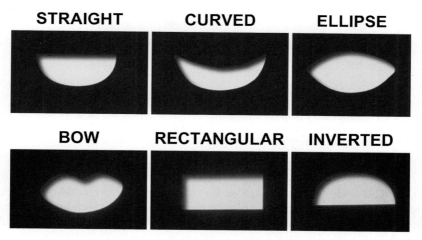

Fig. 5. Smile zone shapes. (*Courtesy of* Nicholas C. Davis, DDS, MAGD, Loma Linda, CA.)

should be firmly anchored to the teeth and underlying alveolar bone. A normal, healthy gingival sulcus should not exceed 3 mm in depth [6].

The gingival contours should be symmetric and the marginal gingival tissues of the maxillary anterior teeth should be located along a horizontal line extending from cuspid to cuspid. Ideally, the laterals reach slightly short of that line (Fig. 7) [5]. It is also acceptable, although not ideal, to have the gingival height of all six anteriors equal in gingival height on the same plane (Fig. 8). In such cases, however, the smile may appear too uniform to be esthetically pleasing. A gingival height of the laterals that is more apical to the centrals and cuspids is considered unattractive (Fig. 9).

The gingival zenith point is the most apical point of the gingival tissues along the long axis of the tooth. Clinical observations along with a review of diagnostic models reveal that this most apical point is located distal to the long axis on the maxillary centrals and cuspids (Fig. 10). The zenith point of the maxillary laterals and the mandibular incisors is coincident with the long axis of these teeth (Fig. 11) [2].

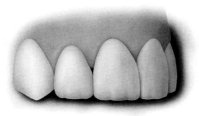

Fig. 6. The black triangle is presenting the cervical embrasure between the central and lateral. (*Courtesy of* American Academy of Cosmetic Dentistry, Madison, WI; with permission.)

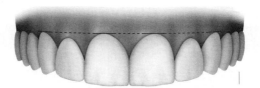

Fig. 7. The gingival margins of the centrals and cuspids are apical to that of the laterals. This appearance is considered more attractive than those shown in Figs. 8 and 9. (*Courtesy of* American Academy of Cosmetic Dentistry, Madison, WI; with permission.)

An attractive smile line is one of the most important features of a pleasing smile. The smile line can be defined as an imaginary line drawn along the incisal edges of the maxillary anterior teeth. In an ideal tooth arrangement, that line should coincide or follow the curvature of the lower lip while smiling (Fig. 12) [9]. Another frame of reference suggests that the centrals are slightly longer than the cuspids. In a reverse smile line, the centrals appear shorter than the cuspids along the incisal plane and create an aged or worn appearance (Fig. 13) [5].

Texts differ on the best height for a maxillary central incisor. One text records the average height from the cementoenamel margin to the incisal edge as 10.5 mm. The importance of tooth length has been recognized and documented in tooth measurement tables recorded by Dr. G.V. Black. In those tables the average height of a maxillary central was noted as 10 mm with the greatest being 12 mm and the least being 8 mm [10]. Another text records the crown height of a maxillary unworn central incisor ranging from 11 to 13 mm with the average height being 12 mm [2].

For esthetic purposes, the height of the central incisors can vary depending upon the incisal display and the influence of the smile line. Other guidelines for determining the dimensions of the maxillary central incisors include the following:

Central incisor length is approximately one sixteenth of the facial height. The ratio of width to height is 4:5 or 0.8:1. In general, the accepted range for the width of the central is 75% to 80% of the height (Fig. 14).

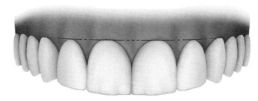

Fig. 8. Similar gingival heights of the six anterior teeth are acceptable although not considered ideal. (*Courtesy of* the American Academy of Cosmetic Dentistry, Madison, WI; with permission.)

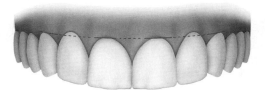

Fig. 9. When the gingival margins of the lateral is apical to that of the centrals, cuspids, or both, the anterior gingival relationship is considered unattractive. (*Courtesy of* American Academy of Cosmetic Dentistry, Madison, WI; with permission.)

> The centrals are most likely too long if they interfere or impinge on the lower lip causing dimpling or entrapment during the formation of the "F" and "V" sounds.
>
> The length of the incisors can also be evaluated using the occlusion. The central is most likely too short or positioned wrong if it is short of a line drawn from the mesial buccal cusp tip of the maxillary first molar and the cusp tip of the cuspid [5].

There are several other considerations when attempting to reestablish normal tooth height, depending on the etiology of the diminished tooth size. Occlusal discrepancies, closed vertical dimension, anterior wear, poor bone and joint relationships, and parafunctional habits can all be considered causative factors. The correct diagnosis leads to the most suitable treatment options for long-term success and stability. In many instances, orthodontic treatment or orthognathic surgery is required before treatment. In other cases, full mouth reconstruction is necessary, often in concert with orthodontic treatment. Cosmetic crown lengthening is another consideration, depending upon conditions or limitations imposed by the patient.

The relative proportions of the maxillary six anterior teeth to each other is another analytical consideration. Many clinicians accept and apply the principles of the Golden Proportion to dentistry. This concept was first mentioned by Lombardi and later developed by Levin [2]. However, the rigidity of this mathematical formula and the many variables among patients have led to many challenges regarding the reliability of this principle. The Golden Proportion suggests an ideal mathematical proportion of 1:1.618. When applied to dentistry, this relates the apparent widths of the maxillary six anterior teeth from a frontal view. The discrepancy between the apparent width

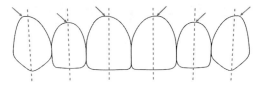

Fig. 10. Gingival shape, zenith point (*arrow*), and longitudinal axis (*dotted lines*). (*Courtesy of* American Academy of Cosmetic Dentistry, Madison, WI; with permission.)

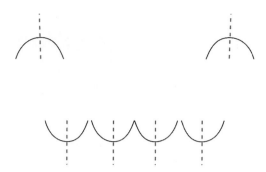

Fig. 11. Gingival shape of maxillary laterals (*upper curved lines*) and mandibular incisors (*lower curved lines*). (*Courtesy of* American Academy of Cosmetic Dentistry, Madison, WI; with permission.)

and actual width is explained by the positioning of these teeth along the curve of the maxillary arch (Fig. 15) [5]. Using this ratio as a guide to direct treatment is a useful tool in esthetic cases for an ideal smile (Fig. 16).

The midline refers to a vertical line formed by the contact of the maxillary central incisors. The midline should be perpendicular to the incisal plane and parallel or coincident to the midline of the face (Fig. 17). Studies have shown that minor discrepancies between facial and dental midlines are acceptable and that in many cases these discrepancies are not noticeable [11]. A canted midline, however, is a more perceptible deviation from the norm [12] and should be avoided.

Several anatomical landmarks can be useful guides to assess the midline of the face as it relates to dental midline. They include the midline of the nose, forehead, interpupillary plane, philtrum, and chin. Some anatomical landmarks may vary in midline accuracy due to variations in genetic structure, such as chin position and the cartilaginous structure of the nose. The philtrum of the lip is considered to be one of the most accurate of these anatomical guideposts as it is always in the center of the face. The exceptions are surgical, accident, and cleft-lip cases. The center of the philtrum

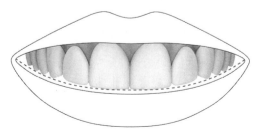

Fig. 12. Ideal smile line. (*Courtesy of* American Academy of Cosmetic Dentistry, Madison, WI; with permission.)

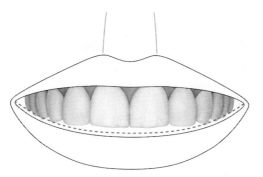

Fig. 13. Reverse smile line. (*Courtesy of* American Academy of Cosmetic Dentistry, Madison, WI; with permission.)

is the center of Cupid's bow and it matches the papilla between the centrals. This places the central papilla directly over the dental midline [5].

A key element in smile design pivots around the midline as it unites the face and its features with dentition and the anterior teeth in particular. From a frontal view, the axial inclination of the anterior teeth tends to incline mesially toward the midline and become more pronounced from the central incisors to the canines. This inclination is least noticeable with the centrals and becomes more pronounced with the laterals and even more so with the canines. The axial inclination of the posterior teeth from the frontal view exhibits the same mesial inclination toward the midline as the cuspid. This also creates a natural visual gradation, making the teeth appear to diminish in size as they progress posteriorly (Fig. 18) [2].

Once again, the lips together with the teeth form another esthetic area that should be considered in smile design. The area between the corners of the mouth during smile formation and the buccal surfaces of the maxillary teeth (particularly the bicuspids and molars) form a space known as the buccal corridor. The greater and more pronounced this negative space becomes, the more these posterior teeth are concealed, restricting the full breadth of the smile (Fig. 19). A full and symmetric buccal corridor is an important element of an esthetic smile. The buccal corridor should not be

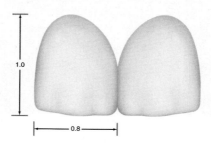

Fig. 14. Proportion of centrals. (*Courtesy of* American Academy of Cosmetic Dentistry, Madison, WI; with permission.)

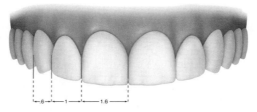

Fig. 15. Golden Proportion. (*Courtesy of* American Academy of Cosmetic Dentistry, Madison, WI; with permission.)

completely eliminated because a hint of negative space imparts a suggestion of depth to the smile [2].

Several factors influence the appearance of the buccal corridor. These factors include the width of the smile and the maxillary arch. Other factors include the tonicity of facial muscles and individual smiling characteristics; the position of the labial surfaces of the maxillary bicuspids; the predominance of the cuspids, particularly at the distal facial line angle; and any discrepancy between the value of the bicuspids and the six anterior teeth. This negative space is often accentuated when smile rejuvenation is limited to the

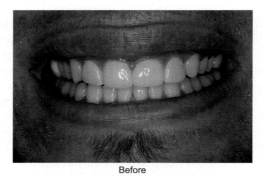

Before

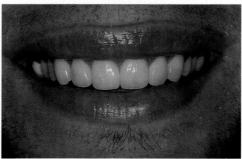

After

Fig. 16. Before (*top*) and after (*bottom*) crown lengthening and application of six porcelain veneers, demonstrating application of proper proportions to the maxillary six anterior teeth. (*Courtesy of* Nicholas C. Davis, DDS, MAGD, Loma Linda, CA.)

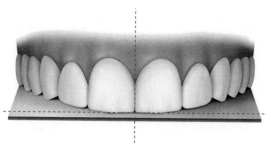

Fig. 17. Midline (*vertical dotted line*). (*Courtesy of* American Academy of Cosmetic Dentistry, Madison, WI; with permission.)

maxillary six anterior teeth and the hue and value of newly restored teeth do not blend with the untreated teeth (Figs. 20A, B). The result is an unwanted exaggeration of the sense of depth, darkness, and the prominence of the buccal corridor [5].

In these posterior segments, the artistic perception of esthetics can be used to alter the typical inclinations to produce an enhanced esthetic affect. Orthodontically up-righting the posterior teeth can help. Also, through cosmetic dentistry to slightly upright the cuspids and the inclination of the posterior segment, the smile can be made to appear wider (Fig. 21). These inclines should not exceed a perfectly vertical orientation. Also, the harmony of having consistent inclines on each of these posterior teeth remains important. These subtle changes can help create a fuller smile that more completely fills the buccal corridor. By up-righting these teeth, the visual foreshortening is diminished. This makes the teeth appear bigger, producing more reflective surfaces for a broader smile, which is in high demand today.

The anatomy of the anterior teeth plays an important role in a natural appearance and the individuality and personality of a smile. Some anterior teeth are flat and some are convex. Some have a square appearance while others have a fan-shaped appearance. These and other distinctive contours give each patient's smile individuality [13]. The labial contour of these teeth should

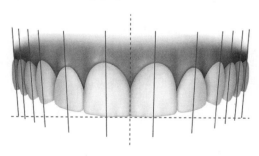

Fig. 18. Axial inclination (*vertical solid lines*). (*Courtesy of* American Academy of Cosmetic Dentistry, Madison, WI; with permission.)

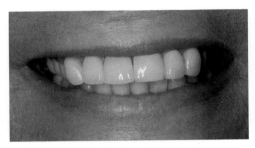

Fig. 19. A dark buccal corridor exists because of the relationship of the anterior teeth with the posterior segments. (*Courtesy of* Nicholas C. Davis, DDS, MAGD, Loma Linda, CA.)

exhibit three planes when viewed from a lateral profile (Figs. 22 and 23) [5]. The surface texture can also add personality to the appearance of the teeth. All of these factors should be considered when restoring teeth in this area.

With ideal anatomy and alignment of these six teeth, an open space is formed between the proximal surfaces of incisal edges from the contact points. This area is called an incisal embrasure. These embrasure spaces terminate at the contact points with the adjacent teeth. The contact areas of both centrals are located at the incisal third of the crowns. Therefore, the incisal embrasure space between the centrals is slight. The contact point between the central and lateral incisor approaches the junction of the middle and incisal thirds of each crown, making it slightly deeper than the junction between the centrals. The contact point of the lateral incisor and the cuspid is approximately at the middle third [10]. Therefore, the incisal embrasure

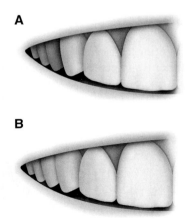

Fig. 20. (*A*) Shadowing effect of the buccal corridor in the posterior segment when compared with an identical diagram (see Fig. 18B) with properly treated hue and value. (*Courtesy of* American Academy of Cosmetic Dentistry, with permission.) (*B*) Properly treated buccal corridor demonstrates uniformity in color and alignment of the anterior segment with the posterior teeth in the smile zone. (*Courtesy of* American Academy of Cosmetic Dentistry, Madison, WI; with permission.)

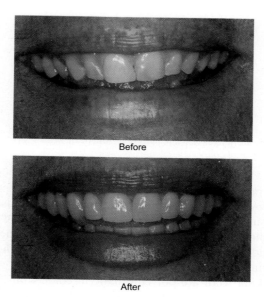

Before

After

Fig. 21. Before and after crown lengthening, bleaching, and application of 10 porcelain veneers. (*Courtesy of* Nicholas C. Davis, DDS, MAGD, Loma Linda, CA.)

spaces of the anterior teeth display a natural and progressive increase in depth from the central to the cuspid (Figs. 24 and 25).

Current trends in smile enhancement have demonstrated an appreciation by the public for whiter teeth. According to a recent American Academy of Cosmetic Dentistry survey of dentists in North America conducted by the Levin Group, "Bleaching/Whitening is the most often requested cosmetic service." Most bleaching experts say the goal is to have the color of the teeth the same as the color of the sclera of the eye. In today's society, however,

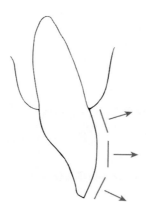

Fig. 22. Labial contour, three planes (cross-sectional view) (*lines perpendicular to arrows*) (*Courtesy of* American Academy of Cosmetic Dentistry, Madison, WI; with permission.)

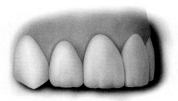

Fig. 23. Labial contour (lateral view). (*Courtesy of* American Academy of Cosmetic Dentistry, Madison, WI; with permission.)

many patients prefer to have their teeth whiter than what is typically found in nature or beyond what bleaching can provide. For this reason, shade selection of cosmetic enhancement cases must be customized to the satisfaction each patient. Counseling the patient on the natural appearance of teeth and general guidelines for shade selection may also be beneficial to meet the patient's expectations of realism.

Natural-looking teeth are polychromatic in color with the body of the tooth fairly uniform in color and the gingival third more rich in chroma. The incisal portion of the tooth typically exhibits a translucency that can vary from bluish-white to blue, gray, orange and other variations. The variations in the coloration of teeth are due to the anatomy of the physical shape and texture of the individual tooth and the basic anatomy of the dentine and enamel structures of the teeth. Typically, hue, chroma, and value are terms used in describing a color or shade of a tooth. Hue refers to the color or shade, such as red, yellow, or blue. Chroma, which refers to the degree of saturation of a color, describes the different shades of the same color (Fig. 26). Value is the term used to describe the relative brightness of a color. It deals with lightness and darkness and is generally measured on a gray scale (Figs. 27 and 28) [5].

An ideal esthetic treatment plan should be minimally invasive, preserving as much of the natural structures as possible. It should also realign the ideal form and function of the teeth and tissues while enhancing the

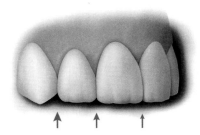

Fig. 24. Incisal embrasures (*arrows*). Size increases progressively from the central to the cuspid. (*Courtesy of* American Academy of Cosmetic Dentistry, Madison, WI; with permission.)

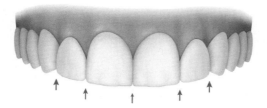

Fig. 25. Incisal embrasures (frontal view) (*arrows*). (*Courtesy of* American Academy of Cosmetic Dentistry, Madison, WI; with permission.)

esthetics and should never compromise the patient's oral health or the stability of his or her teeth.

An ideal esthetic treatment plan attempts to achieve perfection in every way. However, not all patients are willing to accept all the components necessary to achieve that level of perfection. In those cases, when compromises become necessary, it is important to review a range of treatment options in an attempt to create the illusion of the ideal while maintaining a healthy oral environment. A cosmetic dental procedure using porcelain veneers is a common method of creating this illusion.

Conducting a patient interview is helpful in determining the patient's expectations and limitations of treatment. In establishing a treatment plan, goals must be set as a way to measure the success of that treatment. A patient's priority may be to have a bright and esthetic smile first while a dentist's goal should be to achieve oral health first. It is not difficult to achieve both. However, maintaining the patient's enthusiasm through the process may be challenging because the proper sequence of treatment to achieve both stated goals may not be what the patient expects. An understanding of the patient's goals and priorities is helpful for the dentist when the treatment plan is established and presented to the patient.

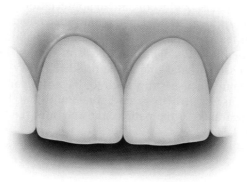

Fig. 26. Color, translucency and color gradient. (*Courtesy of* American Academy of Cosmetic Dentistry, Madison, WI; with permission.)

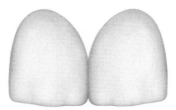

Fig. 27. Both values of the centrals in this example are well matched. (*Courtesy of* American Academy of Cosmetic Dentistry, Madison, WI; with permission.)

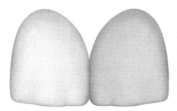

Fig. 28. The value of the central on the right is considered low. (*Courtesy of* American Academy of Cosmetic Dentistry, Madison, WI; with permission.)

This article on smile design did not consider the natural irregularities and random deviations from the norm that contribute to the individuality and beauty of a person's smile. Most beautiful and natural smiles are not necessarily symmetric, uniform in color, or perfect by scientific standards. Consequently, they maintain a natural intrinsic beauty not by the virtue of perfection but rather through the subtle beauty of imperfection. For these reasons, smile design guidelines that use a perfect model as a goal may not necessarily render the most beautiful and natural smile that satisfies both the dentist and patient.

The crafting of an ideal smile requires analyses and evaluations of the face, lips, gingival tissues, and teeth and an appreciation of how they appear collectively. Such an ideal smile depends on the symmetry and balance of facial and dental features. The color, shape, and position of the teeth are all part of the equation. Recognizing that form follows function and that the anterior teeth serve a vital role in the oral health of the patient is paramount. Using a comprehensive approach to diagnosing and treatment planning of esthetic cases can help achieve the smile that best enhances the overall facial appearance of the patient and provides the additional benefit of enhanced oral health.

Acknowledgments

The author thanks the dental team members of the American Academy of Cosmetic Dentistry for their expertise, skills, and help in restoring the cases used in this article and shown in the Criteria Guide publication of the American Academy of Cosmetic Dentistry. The dental team responsible for treating the cases shown in this article are Dr. Michael Gahagan, periodontist, Newport Beach, California; and Stan Okon, Okon Dental Laboratory, El Toro, California.

Appendix 1

Smile analysis form

Smile Analysis

Name: _____   Date: _____
Patients' Dissatisfaction Areas: _____
_____
_____

Patients' Desires /Limitations: _____
_____

FACIAL FORM: SQUARE   OVOID   TAPERING   SQ. TAPERING   **FACIAL PROFILE:**
SMILE ZONE: SHAPE: STRAIGHT   CURVED   BOW   ELLIPSE   RECT.   INVERTED

LIPS: DEPTH:	SHALLOW	AVERAGE	DEEP

THICKNESS: THIN   NORMAL   FULL
UPPER: ☐   ☐   ☐
LOWER: ☐   ☐   ☐

SYMMETRY: ASYMMETRIES
UPPER: NORMAL ☐
LOWER: NORMAL ☐

WIDTH: NARROW   NORMAL   WIDE
BUCCAL CORRIDOR: DARK   NORMAL   FULL
NOTES:_____
_____
_____

GINGIVA:
HEALTH: POOR   FAIR   EXCELLENT
DISPLAY: NONE   PAPILLA   MODERATE   EXCESSIVE
ASYMMETRIES:
NOTES:_____
_____
_____

TEETH:
SMILE LINE LENGTH: LONG   NORMAL   HIGH
SMILE LINE SHAPE: STRAIGHT   CURVED   IRREGULAR
SHADE: WIDTH OF CENTRALS (7.5 - 9.5) _____ MM HEIGHT OF CENTRALS (11 - 13) ____ MM
MIDLINE: CENTERED-   INCLINATION-   LINE ANGLES:
EXISTING RESTORATIONS: _____
_____
_____

NOTES & TX. RECOMMENDATIONS: _____
_____

References

[1] Parramón José M. How to draw heads and portraits. New York: Watson-Guptill Publishing; 1989. p. 14–5.

[2] Rufenacht Claude R. Fundamentals of esthetics. Quintessence Publishing Co.; 1990. p. 73, 80–2, 89, 94, 95, 125–7, 138.

[3] Rufenacht Claude R. Principles of esthetic integration. Quintessence Publishing Co.; 2000. p. 109–11.

[4] Hogarth Burne. Drawing the human head. New York: Watson-Guptill Publishing; 1989. p. 48.

[5] Blitz N, Steel C, Willhite C. Diagnosis and treatment evaluation in cosmetic dentistry—a guide to accreditation criteria. Madison (WI): American Academy of Cosmetic Dentistry; 2001. p. 8–10, 16, 28, 32, 34, 46, 47.

[6] Grant GA, Stern IB, Everett FG. Orban's periodontics. 3rd edition. C.V. Mosby Co; 1968. p. 5–7, 33–5, 387.

[7] Vig RG, Brundo GC. The kinetics of anterior tooth display. J Prosthet Dent 1972;39:502.

[8] Davis Nicholas C. An artistic approach to smile design. Dent Today 1999;18(8):57.

[9] Ahmad I. Geometric considerations in anterior dental esthetics: restorative principles. Pract Periodontics Aesthet Dent 1998;10(7):813–22.

[10] Wheeler RC. A textbook of dental anatomy and physiology. W.B. Saunders; 1965. p. 102, 103, 126, 131, 427.

[11] Miller EC, Bodden WR, Jamison HC. A study of the relationship of the dental midline to the facial midline. J Prosthet Dent 1979;41:657–60.

[12] Kokich Vincent O Jr, Kiyak Asuman H, Shapiro Peter A. Comparing the perception of dentists and lay people to altered dental esthetics. J Esthetic Dent 1999;11:311–24.

[13] Dawson PE. Evaluation, diagnosis and treatment of occlusal problems. The C. V, Mosby Company; 1974. p. 173.

ELSEVIER
SAUNDERS

Dent Clin N Am 51 (2007) 319–331

THE DENTAL
CLINICS
OF NORTH AMERICA

Vital Tooth Whitening

Patricia W. Kihn, DDS, MS[a,b,*]

[a]DENTSPLY International, Inc., Susquehanna Commerce Center,
221 West Philadelphia Street, York, PA 17405-0872, USA
[b]Baltimore College of Dental Surgery, University of Maryland,
Baltimore, MD, USA

Aesthetics of the teeth is of great importance to many patients. Public demand for aesthetic dentistry, including tooth whitening, has increased in recent years. Patient interest in whitening and articles on whitening in popular magazines suggest that tooth color is a significant factor in the attractiveness of a smile. An attractive smile plays a major role in the overall perception of physical attractiveness [1]. Studies confirm the importance of attractiveness on perceived success and self-esteem [2]. Compared with restorative treatment modalities, whitening, also referred to as bleaching, is the most conservative treatment for discolored teeth. This public demand for a whiter smile and improved aesthetics has made tooth whitening a popular and often-requested dental procedure, since it offers a conservative treatment option for discolored teeth. Whitening often enhances the treatment and encourages patients to seek further aesthetic treatment [3].

Successful whitening treatment depends on the correct diagnosis by the practitioner of the type, intensity, and location of the tooth discoloration. It is imperative to determine if the discoloration is extrinsic, which is associated with the absorption of such materials as tea, red wine, some medications, iron salts, tobacco, and foods, onto the surface of the enamel and, in particular, the pellicle coating [4], or intrinsic, where the tooth color is associated with the light-scattering and -absorption properties of the enamel and dentin [5], as seen in tetracycline staining, amelogenesis and dentinogenisis imperfecta, hypoplasia, erythroblastosis fetalis, and porphyria. Additionally, discoloration results from the aging process. As teeth age, more secondary dentin is formed and the more translucent enamel layer thins. The combination of less enamel and darker, opaque dentin creates an older-looking, darker tooth [6]. The practitioner must identify the type of

---

* 932 Castle Pond Drive, York, PA 17402.
E-mail address: kihn1@comcast.net

discoloration, diagnose the cause, and then define the appropriate treatment plan.

Evolution of the technology

Tooth bleaching is not a new technique in dentistry. It was reported more than a century ago [7–11]. In 1916, Adams [12] reported the use of hypochloric acid to treat fluorosis. In 1937, Ames [12a] reported a technique using a mixture of hydrogen peroxide and ethyl ether on cotton, heated with a metal instrument for 30 minutes, and applied over 5 to 25 visits to treat mottled enamel. Younger used this technique in 1942 in 40 children with dental fluorosis. This and similar techniques using concentrated hydrogen peroxide and heat have been accepted treatment since the 1930s [13]. In 1966, the combined use of hydrochloric acid and hydrogen peroxide was promoted to remove brown stain from mottled teeth [14]. In 1970, Cohen and Parkins [15] published a method for whitening tetracycline-discolored dentin of the teeth of young adults treated for cystic fibrosis. This was the first publication indicating that there is chemical penetration of hydrogen peroxide to the dentin to whiten teeth. Previous study concentrated entirely on the removal of extrinsic staining only. In 1976, Nutting and Poe [16] introduced the walking bleach technique, which uses 35% hydrogen peroxide and sodium perborate for whitening nonvital teeth. In 1968, Klusmeier [16a] described a technique using Gly-Oxide (Marion Merrel Dow, Inc., Kansas City, Missouri), a 10% carbamide peroxide oral antiseptic, which he placed in the orthodontic positioners of some patients to improve gingival health. He noted whitened teeth as well as tissue improvement as a result. He switched to Proxigel, which also contained 10% carbamide peroxide, in a custom-fitted night guard in 1972 because the viscosity of the Proxigel allowed it to stay in the tray [6,13].

The first commercially available 10% carbamide peroxide was developed and subsequently marketed by Omni International in 1989 based on the findings of Munro [17], who used a 10% carbamide peroxide solution to control inflammation after root planing in a vacuum-formed plastic splint. He noted whitened teeth. Haywood and Heymann published the first clinical study on tooth whitening using Proxigel in vacuum-formed custom trays. This is the technique known as "night guard vital bleaching" in common use today. Haywood and Heymann [18] conducted laboratory and clinical investigations of this technique and reported it in the literature in 1989. They reported on night guard vital bleaching using 10% carbamide peroxide. The night guard was custom fabricated to hold the whitening gel in contact with the enamel surface.

The dental profession rapidly recognized the benefits of an at-home bleaching agent and it has become a popular method of lightening teeth [19]. The acceptance of this procedure, according to a 1991 use-survey, found 78% of general practitioners perform tooth-whitening procedures with 59% recommending the doctor-prescribed at-home method [20]. In another survey, 9,846 dentists stated using at-home whitening techniques and 79% of those recognized the technique's usefulness and overall clinical success [21]. Ninety-one percent of 8,143 dentists responding to a 1995 Clinical Research Associates (CRA) questionnaire stated that they had used vital tooth bleaching with 79% reporting success and 12% reporting that they were not satisfied with the concept [22].

Many companies followed Omni International's lead, marketing carbamide-peroxide–containing agents directly to consumers. In response to this direct marketing, the Food and Drug Administration issued a statement to manufacturers requiring appropriate safety and efficacy documentation in 1991 [23], and the American Dental Association subsequently developed guidelines for acceptance [24,25]. Currently available peroxide-containing tooth-whitening materials include professionally dispensed and supervised products for use by patients at home, professional-use in-office products, and over-the-counter products for sale directly to consumers.

Mechanism of action

The mechanism of whitening by hydrogen peroxide is not well understood. Hydrogen peroxide whitening generally proceeds via the perhydroxyl anion (HO_2^-). Other conditions can give rise to free radical formation, for example, by hemolytic cleavage of either an O–H bond or O–O bond in hydrogen peroxide to give H + OOH and 2OH (hydroxyl radical), respectively [26]. Under photochemically initiated reactions using light or lasers, the formation of hydroxyl radicals from hydrogen peroxide has been shown to increase [27]. Available literature indicates that teeth are whitened by such materials as hydrogen peroxide and carbamide peroxide by the initial diffusion into and through the enamel to the dentin [28–30]. Hydrogen peroxide is an oxidizing agent that, as it diffuses into the tooth, breaks down to produce unstable free radicals. These unstable free radicals attack organic pigmented molecules in the spaces between the inorganic salts in tooth enamel [6] resulting in smaller, less heavily pigmented constituents. These smaller molecules reflect less light, thus creating a "whitening effect." McCaslin and colleagues [31] demonstrated in vitro that, following external whitening with carbamide peroxide, color change occurred throughout the dentin. Additional studies where dentin specimens were treated using 10% carbamide peroxide, 5.3% hydrogen peroxide and 6% hydrogen peroxide have shown significant reduction in the yellowness of the dentin and an increase in whiteness [32,33]. Sulieman and colleagues [34] showed that significant bleaching of extracted teeth internally stained by black tea was achieved when a 35% hydrogen peroxide gel had been applied.

The color seen in tetracycline-stained teeth is derived from photo-oxidation of tetracycline molecules found within the tooth structures [35]. The mechanism in this case is thought to be by chemical degradation of the unsaturated quinone-type structures found in tetracycline leading to less colored molecules [36]. In some cases, long-term night guard vital bleaching can improve the color of tetracycline-stained teeth [37].

Toxicology

Numerous studies assessing the safety of hydrogen peroxide and carbamide peroxide for tooth whitening indicate that 10% carbamide peroxide, which is equivalent to 3.6% hydrogen peroxide, is safe when applied in the night guard vital bleaching techniques [13,38–40]. Trayless systems in the form of whitening strips, containing 5.3% hydrogen peroxide, and in the form of a paint-on whitening gel, containing 18% carbamide peroxide, are available for use by patients. The concentration is higher than what has been studied to be safe in the previously mentioned studies, but the total contact time is significantly reduced. It is believed that the peroxide dose is no greater than that delivered by tray systems [41]. An in vitro toxicologic study of whitening agents by Li [42] showed fewer or comparable side effects than those with commonly used dental materials, such as eugenol, dentifrices, mouthwashes, and composites. The same study reported that the average amount of tooth-whitening agent used per application is 502 mg. All of this amount swallowed would not exceed 8.37 mg/kg [42], which is below the 10 mg/kg associated with acute toxicity in rats [43]. Peroxides are mutagens and there has been some thought that bleaching should not be recommended to patients who are smokers or heavy drinkers. However, to date, no studies in animals or humans link tooth whitening to oral cancer. The products are regulated by the Food and Drug Administration as cosmetics, not medical devices, and are therefore not subject to Medical Device Reporting requirements. Evidence to date indicates that the safety factor of whitening agents is quite high.

Side effects

The most commonly reported side effects are gingival or mucosal irritation and tooth sensitivity. Other reported side effects include sore throat, temporomandibular dysfunction secondary to long-term tray use, and minor orthodontic tooth movement [44]. Typically, the gingival or mucosal irritation is related to improperly fitted trays, improper or excess application of the gel, and the use of the gel longer than prescribed. The soft tissue irritation noted is usually mild and transient and is resolved shortly after the treatment has ended [45]. Mitigation for soft tissue and throat irritation may require an adjustment of the tray or a reduction of the application period [18]. Mitigation for temporomandibular dysfunction and tooth movement requires use of a thin tray material (0.40 in) for tray fabrication.

Tooth sensitivity is by far the most common side effect reported. Studies have reported that sensitivity occurs in 55% to 75% of the treatment groups. The sensitivity is believed to be the result of the freely diffusible nature of the materials used [46]. Carbamide peroxide decomposes to hydrogen peroxide and urea. Hydrogen peroxide further decomposes to water and oxygen and the urea breaks down to ammonia and carbon dioxide. Some of the by-products pass through the dentinal tubules reaching the pulp, thus causing reversible pulpitis [29,47], resulting in tooth sensitivity. The carrier for many whitening products is glycerin, which absorbs water and causes dehydration during the whitening treatment. This dehydration causes tooth sensitivity [44,48]. The sensitivity related to tooth whitening is generally mild and transient, occurs early in the treatment, and generally decreases as treatment continues with cessation shortly after the treatment ends. Mitigation includes treatment with fluoride gel or a potassium nitrate toothpaste in the tray for 10 to 30 minutes before use of the whitening agent, treatment of the teeth with a desensitizing agent after treatment, and reduction of the number of applications by requiring fewer per day or by requiring applications only every other day. Additionally, use of a potassium nitrate plus fluoride toothpaste 2 weeks before whitening and during the whitening treatment has been suggested as an adjunct therapy for sensitivity management. Although whitening procedures have been reported to induce sensitivity in 55% to 75% of treatment groups, the procedure is well tolerated.

Another consideration with tooth whitening is the effect it has on enamel and dentin. One study found that whitening agents were capable of removing the smear layer from dentin, but produced little or no change in enamel [49]. Additional studies concluded the same result in enamel [46,50] but others have shown changes in porosity and surface morphology of enamel [51–53]. Another study evaluated the effects of take-home whitening systems on enamel surfaces, and suggested that a period of 4 days must elapse before bonding to the enamel of a tooth treated with a peroxide containing whitening agent. However, no delay is necessary if the agent does not contain peroxide [54]. Since the data have produced equivocal results, the current practice is to wait before performing bonding procedures after tooth whitening.

Studies evaluating the effects of home bleaching products on restorative materials have also produced equivocal results. One study found that a home whitening gel significantly reduced the hardness of a hybrid resin composite over a 4-week treatment period. Scanning electron photomicrographs also revealed surface cracking [55]. Whitening agents have been found to adversely affect the color of various restorative materials, with glass ionomers exhibiting the greatest color change [56]. Another investigation found that the shades of two hybrid and one microfill composite were unaffected by two home whitening products [57]. Still another report found no adverse effects from whitening solutions on either the surface texture or color of porcelain, resin composite, amalgam, or gold restorations [49]. Some researchers believe that the tendency for whitening agents to adversely affect restorative materials is related to their pH because greater effects have been noted for products with pH values <5.5. In many instances, restorations are replaced after the whitening treatment at the patient's request or the clinician's recommendation for an improved aesthetic result.

Tooth-whitening systems

A number of methods and approaches for whitening have been described in the literature. There are methods using different whitening agents, concentrations, times of application, product formats, application modes, and light activation methods [6,58,59]. However, three fundamental bleaching approaches exist—dentist-supervised night guard bleaching, in-office or power bleaching, and bleaching with over-the-counter bleaching products [60]. Night guard bleaching typically uses a low level of whitening agent applied to the teeth via a custom-fabricated mouth guard worn at night for at least 2 weeks [6,18,58]. In-office bleaching generally uses high levels of whitening agents (eg, 25%–35% hydrogen-peroxide–containing products) for shorter periods. The whitening gel is applied to the teeth after protection of the soft tissues and the peroxide may be further activated by heat or light [6,58]. The in-office treatment can result in significant whitening after only one treatment visit [6,58] but may require multiple treatment appointments for optimum whitening [61,62]. Over-the-counter products typically contain low levels of whitening agent (eg, 3%–6% hydrogen peroxide), which are self-applied to the teeth via gum shields, strips, or paint-on product formats. These typically require twice-per-day application for up to 2 weeks [63–65].

Professionally dispensed and supervised products for at-home use (take-home systems)

The regimen for take-home systems involves the fabrication of a soft plastic night guard, which may or may not contain reservoirs, to hold the whitening gel in contact with the teeth. The night guard is made from a model of the patient's teeth. Instructions typically call for twice daily treatments of from 30 minutes to 2 hours a day for 2 to 6 weeks, depending on the color of the teeth at the start of treatment [18]. Most of the products also provide the alternative of overnight applications, leaving use up to patient preference. Products are available containing as little as 5% and as much as 36% carbamide peroxide; as well as 6%, 7.5%, 9.5%, 14%, or 15% hydrogen peroxide. Using stronger concentrations of whitening agents will whiten teeth somewhat faster. For example, a quicker two-tab color change has been noted for 10% and 16% carbamide peroxide compared with 5% carbamide peroxide at days 8 and 15 of treatment. However, continuation of the 5% treatment to 3 weeks results in shades that are equivalent to shades achieved after 2-week use of the 10% and 16% treatment regimens. Advantages include lower cost to patient and minimal in-office chair time. Additionally, this technique has the most research and scientific evidence supporting its effectiveness. The major disadvantage is that significant patient compliance is necessary for optimal results. Examples of products for nighttime use include:

Opalescence PF (Ultradent Products), containing 10%, 15%, and 20% carbamide peroxide

Nupro White Gold (DENTSPLY Professional), containing 10% and 15% carbamide peroxide

Nite White Turbo (Discus Dental), containing 6% hydrogen peroxide

PolaNight (Southern Dental Industries), containing 10%, 16%, and 22% carbamide peroxide

Colgate Platinum (Colgate)

Examples of products for daytime use include:

Opalescence PF (Ultradent Products), containing 10%, 15%, and 20% carbamide peroxide

Treswhite (Ultradent Products), containing 9% hydrogen peroxide

Rembrandt XTRA-Comfort (Johnson & Johnson), containing 16%, 22%, and 30% carbamide peroxide

Natural Elegance (Henry Schein), containing 10%, 15%, and 22% carbamide peroxide

JustSmile (JustSmile Whitening Systems), containing 2% to 10% hydrogen peroxide

Perfecta Bravo (Premier Dental Products), containing 9% hydrogen peroxide

PolaDay (Southern Dental Industries), containing 3%, 7.5%, and 9% hydrogen peroxide

Colgate Platinum (Colgate)

In-office treatments

In-office systems typically use a 15%, 30%, or 35% hydrogen peroxide whitening agent, either heated or nonheated, and the recommended use of gingival isolation, either by means of a gingival dam or a gingival paint-on barrier product. The product is applied in the office. Advantages include minimal dependence on patient compliance and immediate visible results, which satisfy patients who want to see quick results. The disadvantages are higher patient cost, the use of chair time, and the requirement of multiple in-office visits to get optimal results and retain them. Examples of products include:

Illumine (DENTSPLY Professional), containing 15% hydrogen peroxide

OfficeWhite (Life-Like Cosmetic Solutions), containing 40% hydrogen peroxide

   Perfection White (Premier Dental Products), containing 35% hydrogen
      peroxide
   Niveous (Shofu Dental), containing 25% hydrogen peroxide
   Opalescence Xtra Boost (Ultradent Products), containing 35% hydrogen
      peroxide

Combination treatment

Combination treatment involves application in the office of a high-con-
centration hydrogen-peroxide agent followed by a professionally dispensed
and supervised product for at-home use for 5 days, often followed by an additional chairside application [66]. Compared with in-office stand-alone
treatment, combination treatments take less time, require fewer office visits,
and cost patients less [67]. The major disadvantage is the need for in-office
chair time. Also, combination treatment is not a one-time treatment, which
patients prefer.

Light-activated treatments

Light-activated treatment involves application in the office of a high-con-
centration hydrogen-peroxide agent, which is then "activated" by plasma-
arc, light-emitting diodes, argon lasers, and metal halide and xenon-halogen
light sources. The theory behind the treatment is that light or heat will speed
the breakdown of the hydrogen peroxide and thus lighten the teeth more
rapidly. The assumed benefit is that the procedure is less time-consuming
while producing faster results. Current studies have produced equivocal results with some touting the benefits [68] while others conclude there is no
benefit [69,70]. Examples of products include

   LaserSmile (Biolase Technology), containing 37% hydrogen peroxide
   ArcBrite (Biotrol), containing 30% hydrogen peroxide
   BriteSmile (BriteSmile), containing 15% hydrogen peroxide
   Rembrandt Lightening Plus (Johnson & Johnson), containing 35%
      hydrogen peroxide
   Zoom (Discus Dental), containing 20% hydrogen peroxide
   LumaWhite Plus (LumaLite), containing 35% hydrogen peroxide

Over-the-counter treatments

Over-the-counter treatments include dentifrices, whitening strips, paint-
on brush applications, and whitening kits complete with a preformed or
semimolded tray. The toothpastes marketed as whitening products typically
contain a mild abrasive to remove surface stains and some contain a minimal
amount of peroxide. The exposure time to the toothpaste is minimal. Therefore any potential whitening in minimal [71]. Whitening strips use 6.5% hydrogen peroxide and the paint-on brush application uses 18% carbamide
peroxide as the whitening agent. Contact time is significantly reduced as

compared with professionally prescribed products. Therefore, whitening strips and paint-on brush applications must be used longer to obtain similar results to those from the professionally prescribed products. Minimal research exists on these products and, because they can be bought and used indiscriminately by patients, the risk of inappropriate use is high. Long-term risks have yet to be determined [72]. These methods are excellent for maintaining already whitened teeth and are a good option for patients who cannot afford the professionally prescribed products or who do not have time for multiple office visits [73].

The whitening kits with supplied tray and whitening agent present patient problems in that the trays are not custom fitted and the formulations may be variable as compared with the products for sale to dentists [74]. Results obtained from these products vary. Examples of products include Crest White-strips (Proctor & Gamble), containing 6.5% hydrogen peroxide; and Simply-White Whitening Gel (Colgate), containing 5.9% hydrogen peroxide.

Efficacy

Vital night guard whitening using 10% carbamide peroxide has been in use for close to 20 years and has been the most extensively researched method for tooth whitening. It has been shown to be effective for lightening primary teeth discolored by trauma [75]; lightening tetracycline-stained teeth [37]; removing brown stain, including fluorosis stain [76]; and lightening teeth stained by nicotine. It will not, however, change the color of roots of teeth, and this must be taken into consideration in the patient's treatment plan. The teeth get lighter through the process and reach a maximum lightness regardless of the concentration of the agent or contact time used. Once treatment is completed, the teeth will rebound by approximately a half shade, probably due to the complete rehydration of the teeth. There is minimal information regarding retention. Retention studies reported satisfactory shade retention in 82% of the cases treated at 47 months posttreatment [77,78] and long-term retention of the shade change at a satisfactory level without re-treatment for 10 years posttreatment in at least 43% of the cases [77,79].

Unanswered questions

Areas of further research with regard to whitening include elucidation of the true mechanism of action, the nature and composition of colored materials naturally found within the dental hard tissues, and the mechanistic effects of peroxide on these structures. Joiner [80] believes this is necessary research if the chemical mechanistic aspects of tooth bleaching are to be resolved. There is much research around whitening, but most is reported on use of the 10% carbamide peroxide products. Therefore further research of the effects and dose on outcomes of the higher-concentration products is warranted. Further information is required regarding how long the whitening effect lasts, at what point and what patient factors lead to rebound, and what is an appropriate recommendation for the maintenance of whitening. There are a number of approaches to measuring color change and research for standardization to measure color change would remove the human variable and provide more reliable results for comparison of products. Current information regarding the effects on enamel and dentin is controversial and additional information is needed on the effects to provide good recommendations to practitioners regarding placement of composite resins after whitening. Current information regarding whether the use of light and heat to activate the whitening is necessary is also controversial and further research is needed in this area to elucidate if this is really beneficial to the whitening process and patients or just a marketing ploy. Lastly, more research is needed to provide better and more consistent management of tooth sensitivity, which can be quite significant, or to find products or additives to products to mitigate the sensitivity during treatment.

Summary

The typical result of treatment is a whiter appearance of the teeth, which reduces the aged look patients may have as a result of more yellow, darker teeth. This whiter appearance often leads to a heightened awareness of other problems with dentition and a desire for further treatment. The dentist can play an active role in encouraging patients and educating them about choices for tooth whitening and in providing them the best treatment option. To that end, dentists who provide this service need to educate themselves to be able to effectively inform their patients of the benefits and risks of the different options for whitening based on as much scientific evidence as possible, of additional treatment that may be necessary after whitening, and of the cost/benefit ratio of the treatment. Vital tooth whitening, when administered correctly, is by all accounts one of the safest, most conservative, least expensive, and most effective aesthetic procedures currently available to patients.

References

[1] Patzer GL. Reality of physical attractiveness. J Esthet Dent 1994;6:35–58.
[2] Dunn J. Dentist prescribed home bleaching: current status. Compend Contin Educ Dent 1998;19(8):760–4.
[3] Barghi N. Making a clinical decision for vital tooth bleaching: at-home or in-office? Compend Contin Educ Dent 1998;19(8):831–8.
[4] Joiner A, Jones NM, Raven SJ. Investigation of factors influencing stain formation utilizing an in situ model. Adv dent Res 1995;9:471–6.

[5] Ten Bosch JJ, Coops JC. Tooth color and reflectance as related to tooth scattering and enamel hardness. J Dent Res 1995;74:373–80.

[6] Goldstein RE, Garber DA. Complete dental bleaching. Chicago: Quintessence Publishing; 1995. p. 73–4.

[7] Fitch CP. Etiology of the discoloration of teeth. Dent Cosmos 1861;3(3):133–6.

[8] White JD. Bleaching. Dent Register West 1861;15:576–7.

[9] Harlan AW. Hydrogen dioxide (in the treatment of alveolar abscess, pyorrhea and the bleaching of teeth). Dent Cosmos 1882;24(10):515–23.

[10] Westlake A. Bleaching teeth by electricity. Am J Dent 1895;29:101.

[11] Burchard HH. A textbook of dental pathology and therapeutics. Philadelphia: Lea & Febiger; 1898. p. 258–9.

[12] Adams TC. Enamel color modifications by controlled hydrochloric acid pumice abrasion: a review with case summaries. J Indian Dent Assoc 1987;66(5):23–6.

[12a] Ames JW. Removing stains from mottled enamel. JADA and Dent Cosmos 1937;24: 1674–7.

[13] Li Y. Biological properties of peroxide-containing tooth whiteners. Food Chem Toxicol 1996;34:887–904.

[14] McInnes J. Removing brown stain from teeth. Ariz Dent J 1966;12(4):13–45.

[15] Cohen S, Parkins FM. Bleaching tetracycline-stained vital teeth. Oral Surg Oral Med Oral Pathol 1970;29(3):465–71.

[16] Nutting EB, Poe GS. Chemical bleaching of discolored endodontically treated teeth. Dent Clin North Am 1967;10:655–62.

[16a] Goldstein RE, Garber DA. Complete dental bleaching. Chicago: Quintessence Publishing; 1995. p. 73–4.

[17] Darnell DH, Moore WC. Vital tooth bleaching: the White and Brite technique. Compend Contin Educ Dent 1990;11:86–94.

[18] Haywood VB, Heymann HO. Night guard vital bleaching. Quintessence Int 1989;20:173–6.

[19] Christensen G, Christensen R. Tooth bleaching, home-use products. Clinical Research Associates Newsletter 1989;13(12):1–3.

[20] Reis-Schmidt T, editor. Status of whitening examined prior to FDA action. Dent Prod Reports 1991;(25)1:86–89.

[21] Christensen G, Christensen R. Home-use bleaching survey. Clinical Research Associates Newsletter 1991;15(2):2–3.

[22] Christensen G, Christensen R. Home-use bleaching survey. Clinical Research Associates Newsletter 1995;19(10):1.

[23] Berry J. FDA says whiteners are drugs. ADA News 1991;22(18): 1, 6, 7.

[24] Council on Dental Therapeutics. Guidelines for acceptance of peroxide-containing oral hygiene products. J Am Dent Assoc 1994;125:1140–2.

[25] American Dental Association Council on Scientific Affairs. Acceptance program guidelines: home use tooth whitening products. Chicago: American Dental Association; 1998.

[26] In: Howe-Grant M. editor. Encyclopedia of chemical technology, 4th edition, vol. 4. New York: John Wiley and Sons; 1992;290–91.

[27] Kashima-Tanaka M, Tsujimoto Y, Kawamoto K, et al. Generation of free radicals and/or active oxygen by light or laser irradiation of hydrogen peroxide or sodium hypochlorite. J Endod 2003;29:141–3.

[28] Bowles WH, Ugwuneri Z. Pulp chamber penetration by hydrogen peroxide following vital bleaching procedures. J Endod 1987;13(8):375–7.

[29] Bowles WH, Thompson LR. Vital bleaching: the effect of heat and hydrogen peroxide on pulpal enzymes. J Endod 1986;12(3):108–12.

[30] Fuss Z, Szajkis S, Tagger M. Tubular permeability to calcium hydroxide and to bleaching agents. J Endod 1989;15(8):362–4.

[31] McCaslin AJ, Haywood VB, Potter BJ, et al. Assessing dentin color changes from night-guard vital bleaching. J Am Dent Assoc 1999;130:1485–90.

[32] Joiner A, Thakker G, Cooper Y. Evaluation of a 6% hydrogen peroxide tooth whitening gel on enamel and dentin microhardness in vitro. J Dent 2004;32(Suppl 1):27–34.

[33] White DJ, Kozak KM, Zoladz JR, et al. Effects of tooth-whitening gels on enamel and dentin ultrastructure-a confocal laser scanning microscopy pilot study. Compend Contin Educ Dent 2000;21(Suppl 29):S29–34.

[34] Sulieman M, Addy M, Macdonald E, et al. The bleaching depth of a 35% hydrogen peroxide based in-office product: a study in vitro. J Dent 2005;33:33–40.

[35] Mello HS. The mechanism of tetracycline staining in primary and permanent teeth. J Dent Child 1967;34:478–87.

[36] Feinman RA, Madray G, Yarborough D. Chemical, optical, and physiologic mechanisms of bleaching products: a review. Pract Periodontics Aesthet Dent 1991;3:32–6.

[37] Leonard RH, Haywood VB, Caplan DJ, et al. Nightguard vital bleaching of tetracycline-stained teeth: 90 months post treatment. J Esthet and Rest Dent 2003;15:142–53.

[38] Haywood VB. Considerations and variations of dentist-prescribed, home-applied vital tooth-bleaching technique. Compend Contin Educ Dent 1994;15(Suppl 17):616–21.

[39] Marshall MV, Cancro LP, Fischman SL. Hydrogen peroxide: a review of its use in dentistry. J Periodontol 1995;66:786–96.

[40] Li Y. Peroxide-containing tooth whiteners: an update on safety. Compend Contin Educ Dent 2000;21(Suppl 28):4–9.

[41] Collins LZ, Maggio B, Gallagher A, et al. Safety evaluation of a novel whitening gel, containing 6% hydrogen peroxide and a commercially available gel containing 18% carbamide peroxide in an exaggerated use clinical study. J Dent 2004;32:47–50.

[42] Li Y. Toxicological considerations of tooth bleaching using peroxide containing agents. J Am Dent Assoc 1997;128(Suppl):31S–6S.

[43] Dahl JE, Bechler R. Acute toxicity of carbamide peroxide and commercially available tooth-bleaching agent in rats. J Dent Res 1995;74(2):710–4.

[44] Pohjola R, Browning WD, Hackman ST, et al. Sensitivity and tooth whitening agents. J Esthet Restor Dent 2002;14(2):85–91.

[45] Haywood VB, Leonard RH, Chauncy NF, et al. Effectiveness, side effects and long-term status of nightguard vital bleaching. J Am Dent Assoc 1994;125(9):1219–26.

[46] Haywood VB, Leech T, Heymann HO, et al. Nightguard vital bleaching: effects on enamel surface texture and diffusion. Quintessence Int 1990;21:801–4.

[47] Gokay O, Tuncbilek M, Ertan P. Penetration of the pulp chamber by carbamide peroxide bleaching agents on teeth restored with composite resin. J Oral Rehabil 2000;27(5):428–31.

[48] Leonard RH, Haywood VB, Phillips C. Risk factors for developing tooth sensitivity and gingival irritation associated with nightguard vital bleaching. Quintessence Int 1997; 28(8):527–34.

[49] Hunsaker KJ, Christensen GJ. Tooth bleaching chemicals—influence on teeth and restorations [abstract]. J Dent Res 1990;69:303.

[50] Haywood VB, Houck V, Heymann HO. Night guard vital bleaching: effects of varying pH solutions on enamel surface texture and color change. Quintessence Int 1991;22:775–82.

[51] Ben-Amar A, Liberman R, Gorfil C, et al. Effect of mouthguard bleaching on enamel surface. Am J Dent 1995;8:29–32.

[52] Bitter NC. A scanning electron microscopy study of the long-term effect of bleaching agents on enamel: a preliminary report. J Prosthet Dent 1992;67:852–5.

[53] Bitter NC. A scanning electron microscope study of the long-term effect of bleaching agents on the enamel surface in vivo. Gen Dent 1998;46:84–8.

[54] MacKay M, Perry R, Swift E, et al. Effects of the two home bleaching systems on enamel surfaces. J Dent Res 1997;76(spec. iss.) [abstract 1405].

[55] Bailey SJ, Swift EJ. Effects of home bleaching products on resin composites [abstract]. J Dent Res 1991;70:570.

[56] Kao EC, Peng P, Johnson WM. Color changes of teeth and restorative materials exposed to bleaching agents [abstract]. J Dent Res 1991;70:570.

[57] Monaghan P, Lee E, Lautenschlager EP. At home, vital bleaching effects on composite resin color [abstract]. J Dent Res 1997;70:570.

[58] Kugel G, Ferreira S. The art and science of tooth whitening. Inside Dentistry 2006;2(7): 84, 86–9.

[59] Sulieman M. An overview of bleaching techniques. 1. History, chemistry, safety and legal aspects. Dent Update 2004;31:608–16.

[60] Heymann HO. Tooth whitening: facts and fallacies. Br Dent J 2005;198:5–14.

[61] Shethri SA, Matis BA, Cochran MA, et al. A clinical evaluation of two in-office bleaching products. Oper Dent 2003;28:488–95.

[62] Sulieman M. An overview of bleaching techniques. 3. In surgery or power bleaching. Dent Update 2005;32:101–8.

[63] Gerlach RW. Whitening paradigms 1 year later: introduction of a novel professional tooth-bleaching system. Compend Contin Educ Dent 2002;23(Suppl 1A):4–8.

[64] Slezak B, Santarpia P, Xu T, et al. Safety profile of a new liquid whitening gel. Compend Contin Educ Dent 2002;23(Suppl 1):S4–11.

[65] Collins LZ, Maggio B, Liebman J, et al. Clinical evaluation of a novel whitening gel, containing 6% hydrogen peroxide and a standard fluoride toothpaste. J Dent 2004;32(Suppl 1): 13–7.

[66] Kugel G, Perry RD, Hoang E, et al. Effective tooth bleaching in 5 days: using a combined in-office and at-home bleaching system. Compend Contin Educ Dent 1997;18(4):378–83.

[67] Garber DA. Dentist-monitored bleaching: a discussion of combination and laser bleaching. J Am Dent Assoc 1997;128(Suppl):26S–30S.

[68] Tavares M, Stultz J, Newman M, et al. Light augments tooth whitening with peroxide. J Am Dent Assoc 2003;134(2):167–75.

[69] Hein DK, Ploeger BJ, Hartup JK, et al. In office vital tooth bleaching—what do lights add? Compend Contin Educ Dent 2003;24(4A):340–52.

[70] Papathanasiou A, Kastali S, Perry RD, et al. Clinical evaluation of a 35% hydrogen peroxide in-office whitening system. Compend Contin Educ Dent 2002;23(4):335–8.

[71] Donly KJ, Donly AS, Baharloo L, et al. Tooth whitening in children. Compend Contin Educ Dent 2002;23(1A):22–8.

[72] Li Y. The safety of peroxide-containing at-home whiteners. Compend Contin Educ Dent 2003;24(4A):384–9.

[73] Kugel G. Nontray whitening. Compend Contin Educ Dent 2000;21(6):524–8.

[74] Kugel G. Over-the-counter tooth-whitening systems. Compend Contin Educ Dent 2003; 24(4A):376–83.

[75] Brantley DH, Barnes KP, Haywood VB. Bleaching primary teeth with 10% carbamide peroxide. Pediatr Dent 2001;23(6):514–6.

[76] Haywood VB, Leonard RH. Nightguard vital bleaching removes brown discoloration for 7 years: a case report. Quintessence Int 1998;29(7):450–1.

[77] Leonard RH Jr. Long-term treatment results with night guard vital bleaching. Compend Contin Educ Dent 2003;24(4A):364–74.

[78] Ritter AV, Leonard RH Jr, St Georges AJ, et al. Safety and stability of night guard vital bleaching: 9 to 12 years post-treatment. J Esthet Restor Dent 2002;14(5):275–85.

[79] Leonard RH Jr, Bentley C, Eagle JC, et al. Nightguard vital bleaching: a long term study on efficacy, shade retention, side effects and patient's perceptions. J Esthet Restor Dent 2001; 13(6):357–69.

[80] Joiner A. The bleaching of teeth: a review of the literature. J Dent 2006;34:412–9.

THE DENTAL
CLINICS
OF NORTH AMERICA

Dent Clin N Am 51 (2007) 333–357

New Developments in Dental Adhesion

Jorge Perdigão, DMD, MS, PhD

*Division of Operative Dentistry, Department of Restorative Sciences,
University of Minnesota, 8-450 Moos Health Sciences Tower,
515 Delaware Street SE, Minneapolis, MN 55455, USA*

Adhesion or bonding is the process of forming an adhesive joint, which consists of two substrates joined together. In dentistry, the adherend is the substrate to which the adhesive—enamel and dentin, rarely cementum— is applied. Dental adhesives are solutions of resin monomers that join a restorative material with a dental substrate after the monomers set by polymerization. While most adhesive joints involve only two interfaces, dental adhesive joints may be more complex such as the enamel–adhesive–composite–adhesive–porcelain interface formed when a clinician bonds a porcelain restoration (Fig. 1). A bonded composite restoration is another example of a complex adhesive joint.

In 1955, Buonocore [1] reported the use of 85% phosphoric acid to improve the retention of an acrylic resin on enamel. The micromechanical nature of the interaction of dental adhesives with enamel is a result of the infiltration of resin monomers into the microporosities left by the acid dissolution of enamel and subsequent enveloping of the exposed hydroxyapatite crystals with the polymerized monomers within the pores on the enamel surface [2].

The ultimate goal of a bonded restoration is to attain an intimate adaptation of the restorative material with the dental substrate [3]. This task is difficult to achieve as the bonding process for enamel is different from that for dentin. That is, dentin is more humid and more organic than enamel [4]. While enamel is composed of 96% hydroxyapatite (mineral) by weight, dentin contains a significant amount of water and organic material, mainly type-I collagen [5]. This humid and organic nature of dentin makes bonding to this hard tissue extremely difficult.

When tooth structure is cut with a bur or other instrument, the residual components form a "smear layer" of debris on the surface [6]. This debris

E-mail address: perdi001@umn.edu

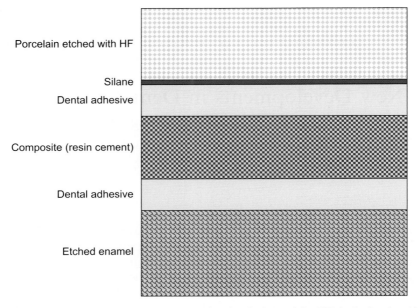

Porcelain etched with HF

Silane
Dental adhesive

Composite (resin cement)

Dental adhesive

Etched enamel

Fig. 1. Adhesive joint formed between enamel and etched porcelain. HF, hydrofluoric acid.

forms a uniform coating on enamel and dentin and plugs the entrance of the dentinal tubules, reducing the permeability of dentin (Fig. 2). The smear layer is porous and permeable as a result of submicron channels that allow the dentinal fluid to pass through [4]. The basic composition of the smear layer is hydroxyapatite and altered collagen with an external surface formed by gellike denatured collagen [7]. The morphology of the smear layer is determined to a large extent by the type of instrument that creates it and by the site of dentin where it is formed [8,9].

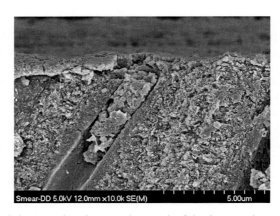

Fig. 2. Field emission scanning electron micrograph of dentin smear layer and smear plug.

As the smear layer constitutes a true physical barrier, it must be dissolved or made permeable so the monomers in the adhesives can contact the dentin surface directly. In spite of different classifications of adhesive systems, the current adhesion strategies depend exclusively on how dental adhesives interact with this smear layer. One strategy involves etch-and-rinse adhesives, which remove the smear layer and superficial hydroxyapatite through etching with a separate acid gel (Fig. 3). The second strategy involves self-etch adhesives, which make the smear layer permeable without removing it completely (Figs. 4 and 5). Fig. 6 summarizes the current bonding strategies.

Etch-and-rinse strategy

With the etch-and-rinse strategy, dentin and enamel are treated with an acid gel (commonly phosphoric acid) to remove the smear layer and demineralize the most superficial hydroxyapatite crystals (Fig. 7). Following this chemical etching, a mixture of resin monomers (primer/adhesive) dissolved in an organic solvent is applied to infiltrate etched dentin [10]. The resin monomers permeate the water-filled spaces between adjacent dentin collagen fibers that used to be occupied by hydroxyapatite crystals. This infiltration results in a hybrid tissue composed of collagen, resin, residual hydroxyapatite, and traces of water (see Fig. 3) known as the resin–dentin interdiffusion zone, first described in 1982 as the hybrid layer [11]. This intimate micromechanical entanglement of resin monomers with etched dentin

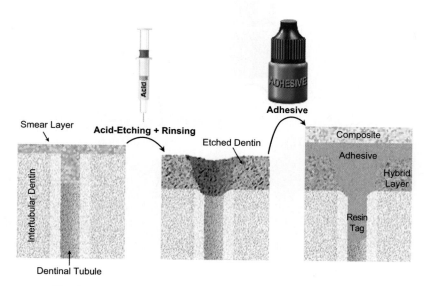

Fig. 3. Interaction of one-bottle etch-and-rinse adhesives with dentin.

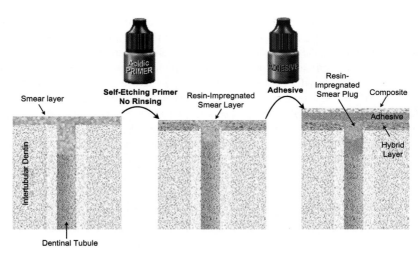

Fig. 4. Interaction of two-bottle self-etch adhesives with dentin.

may result in decreased postoperative sensitivity, may make for a better marginal fit, and may even act as an elastic buffer that compensates for the polymerization shrinkage stress during contraction of the restorative composite [12–14].

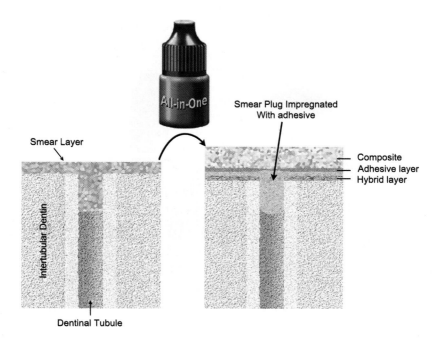

Fig. 5. Interaction of all-in-one self-etch adhesives with dentin.

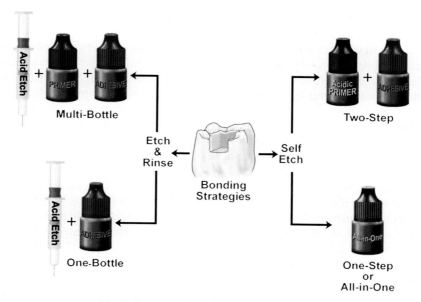

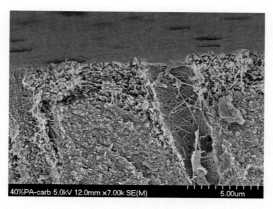

Fig. 6. Summary of current adhesion strategies.

Self-etch strategy

The latest development in dental adhesion is based on simplification and reduced application time. These self-etch (nonrinsing) adhesives do not require a separate acid-etch step as they condition and prime enamel and dentin simultaneously by infiltrating and partially dissolving the smear layer

Fig. 7. Field emission scanning electron micrograph of dentin etched with 40% phosphoric acid for 15 seconds. Note the collagen fibers deprived from hydroxyapatite crystals as a result of acid demineralization. The more intense decalcification around the peritubular area may be a result of both the high mineral content of the peritubular region and the easier penetration of the acid through the tubular lumen.

and hydroxyapatite to generate a hybrid zone that incorporates minerals and the smear layer [15].

The first self-etch nonrinsing adhesives were composed of two solutions, an acidic primer and a bonding resin (see Fig. 4). Recently, many clinicians have shifted to one-step self-etch systems (also named all-in-one adhesives) in which manufacturers have attempted to incorporate all the primary components of an adhesive system (etchant, primer, and bonding resin) into a single solution (see Fig. 5). Both the acidic primer of two-step self-etch adhesives and the all-in-one solution are composed of aqueous mixtures of acidic functional monomers, generally phosphoric-acid or carboxylic-acid esters, with a pH higher than that of phosphoric acid gels [16]. Water is an essential component of self-etch adhesives as it participates in the ionization of the acidic moieties.

All-in-one adhesives are user-friendly in that fewer steps are required for the bonding protocol. The elimination of separate etching and rinsing steps simplified the bonding technique, making these systems more popular in daily practice [17].

Self-etch adhesives differ in their aggressiveness. Therefore they are classified in three categories according to acidity: mild, moderate, and aggressive [16,18]. Because self-etch adhesives are not as aggressive as the phosphoric-acid gel in etch-and-rinse adhesives, most do not remove the smear layer (Fig. 8). Adper Prompt L-Pop (3M ESPE) is considered an aggressive self-etch adhesive (pH = 0.9–1.0), while other all-in-one adhesives, such as Clearfil S3 Bond, iBond, and G-Bond, are mild or moderate (pH > 1.5) (Table 1) [19–22].

Enamel bonding with self-etch adhesives

The enamel bond strengths of the earliest self-etch adhesives were lower than those associated with adhesives that rely on a separate etching step [23].

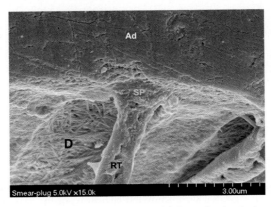

Fig. 8. Field emission scanning electron micrograph of a resin–dentin interface formed with Clearfil S³ Bond (Kuraray). The neck of the resin tag contains residual smear layer particles. Ad, adhesive; D, dentin; RT, resin tag; SP, resin-impregnated smear plug.

Table 1
pH[a] of self-etch adhesives

Adhesive (manufacturer)	pH
AdheSE (Ivoclar Vivadent)	1.7
Adper Prompt L-Pop (3M ESPE)	0.9–1.0
Clearfil S³ Bond (Kuraray)	2.4
Clearfil SE Bond (Kuraray)	1.8
iBond (Heraeus Kulzer)	2.2
Xeno IV (Dentsply Caulk)	2.5

[a] pH of 35% silica-thickened phosphoric-acid gel = 0–0.4.
Data from Refs. [19–22].

Because of their higher pH, two-step self-etch adhesives result in shallower enamel demineralization compared with that of phosphoric acid [16,23]. Nevertheless, roughening of enamel to remove prismless enamel improves the enamel-bonding ability of self-etch adhesives [24]. A separate phosphoric-acid enamel-etching step also enhances the efficacy of self-etch adhesives [25]. Two-step self-etch adhesives bond at an acceptable level to normal dentin and to ground enamel in vitro [26–28]. Conversely, two-step self-etch materials may not bond as well to intact enamel and sclerotic dentin [16,24,29,30].

All-in-one self-etch systems are not as acidic as the phosphoric acid used with the etch-and-rinse adhesives [2]. This characteristic has raised concerns about the performance of all-in-one self-etch systems on intact enamel (Fig. 9). Several in vitro investigations have reported low resin–enamel bond strength of all-in-one self-etch materials [15,26,30,31]. Grinding the enamel during a bevel or cavity preparation, for instance, makes the substrate more receptive for bonding with all-in-one self-etch systems [31,32].

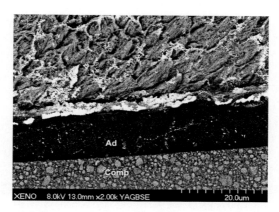

Fig. 9. Backscattered field emission scanning electron micrograph of resin–enamel interface formed by Xeno IV (Dentsply). The restorative material used was Filtek Z250 (3M ESPE). Intense silver deposits at the resin–enamel interface (*asterisks*) denote intense enamel leakage. Ad, adhesive; Comp, composite restoration.

Despite the increased popularity of self-etch adhesives, etching with phosphoric acid is still considered the golden standard against which new materials are tested [27].

Dentin bonding with self-etch adhesives

In spite of their user-friendliness and low technique sensitivity, all-in-one adhesives have resulted in low bonding effectiveness in vitro [15,26,30] while their clinical reliability has often been questioned. Another drawback associated with all-in-one adhesives is their behavior as semipermeable membranes. These materials allow the movement of water across the bonded interface, which potentially leads to hydrolytic degradation (Fig. 10) [31,32].

Consistent information regarding the durability of self-etch adhesives when applied on dentin is available in the literature [28,33,34]. Although high early resin–dentin bond-strength values may be achieved with self-etch adhesives, their bonding effectiveness over time is disappointing [28,33,34]. Because of the high hydrophilic nature of the acidic monomers and the high water concentration required for ionization of the acidic monomers in all-in-one self-etch solutions, these materials are likely to have resin–enamel bonds compromised over time. An inadequate resin penetration into tooth substrates may result in accelerated degradation of the structure of the bonding interface [30]. As polymerization shrinkage stresses the bonding interface, dentin adhesives that do not resist these stresses result in low bond strengths, marginal gaps, recurrent caries, and pulpal irritation [33,35].

For some all-in-one adhesives, performance may depend on the application method, as the number of coats recommended by the manufacturer may not suffice [30,36]. All-in-one adhesives have resulted in a wide range of dentin bond strengths [30,36,37]. Application of the all-in-one adhesive in multiple layers may result in higher bond strengths [37,38] and better

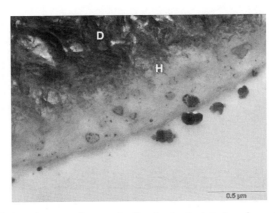

Fig. 10. Transmission electron micrograph of resin–dentin interface formed with Clearfil S3 Bond (Kuraray). Deposits of silver grains may correspond to areas of residual water. D, dentin; H, hybrid layer.

infiltration into the hybrid layer [38]. One manufacturer recommends rubbing the adhesive continuously for 15 seconds, followed by the application of a second coat after gentle air-drying and curing the first coat. This second coat prevents the formation of dry spots on the dentin surface and may result in better impregnation of the monomers into the hybrid layer, as observed in Figs. 11 and 12.

Low enamel and dentin bond strengths have been reported when acetone-based all-in-one adhesives are applied as per manufacturer's directions [33,37]. These adhesives result in severe enamel microleakage following thermal stresses [39,40]. When applied to one-surface occlusal preparations, one of the most popular acetone-based all-in-one adhesives is not able to withstand polymerization shrinkage stresses nor thermocycling, resulting in a high percentage of pretesting debonds [33]. Several mechanisms may account for this poor performance as compared with adhesives with different solvents. The magnitude of dentin bond strengths depends on the degree of infiltration of the resin monomers into the collagen pretreated with an acidic conditioner or with phosphoric acid [41]. The author's electron microscopy analyses (Figs. 13 and 14) have demonstrated that acetone-based all-in-one adhesives result in a hybrid layer 0.2 to 0.5 μm thick, interfacial gaps, and limited resin penetration into the dentinal tubules. It is known that hybrid layers are particularly susceptible to degradation when the cavo-surface margins are not in enamel [42]. The degradation of the dentin bonding interface is caused by the availability of exposed collagen fibrils at the base of hybrid layer [43] or by hydrolytic degradation of resin components in the hybrid layer [28,43–45]. Water can also infiltrate and plasticize

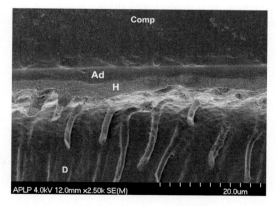

Fig. 11. Field emission scanning electron micrograph of the dentin hybridization formed upon application of two coats of Adper Prompt L-Pop. Note the infiltration of the material into the dentin tubules and the absence of interfacial gaps. When Adper Prompt L-Pop is applied in one coat, a separation gap forms between the adhesive and the hybrid layer (not shown). Ad, adhesive; Comp, composite restoration; D, dentin; H, hybrid layer.

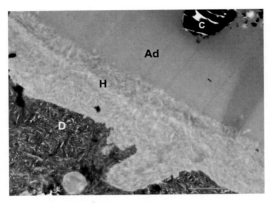

Fig. 12. Transmission electron micrograph of the dentin hybridization formed upon application of two coats of Adper Prompt L-Pop (3M ESPE). Note the reticular morphology of the hybrid layer corresponding to the resin embedding of the collagen fibers. Ad, adhesive; C, composite particle; D, dentin; H, hybrid layer.

the resin matrix, which decreases the mechanical properties of the polymer [46].

Other factors may play a role in the weak bonding performance of acetone-containing all-in-one adhesives. Porosities (or blisters) occur at the enamel and dentin bonding interfaces because most all-in-one adhesives behave as semipermeable membranes [31,33,47–49]. These porosities may be a result of water accumulation either caused by an osmotic gradient or by monomer–solvent phase separation upon evaporation of the acetone [21,49]. The number and size of these blisters may also depend on the intensity of the air-drying step [47].

High hydrophilicity, and consequent higher water sorption, has been reported associated with another acetone-based all-in-one adhesive containing

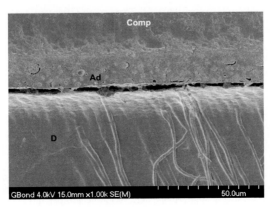

Fig. 13. Field emission scanning electron micrograph of a resin–dentin interface formed with G-Bond (GC America). Ad, adhesive; Comp, composite restoration; D, dentin.

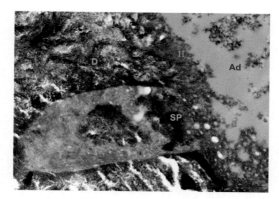

Fig. 14. Transmission electron micrograph of a resin–dentin interface formed with G-Bond (GC America) Asterisks indicate residual smear particles. Ad, adhesive; D, dentin; H, hybrid layer; SP, smear plug; T, resin tag.

a poly-phosphate molecule, dipentaerythritol penta-acrylate phosphate [50]. The adhesive may undergo a substantial reduction in elastic modulus after water sorption, due to the plasticizing effect of water [50]. If the adhesive has been plasticized by water, the restoration will likely fail when a load is applied on the surface because the stresses cannot be transferred across the adhesive joint. Another factor that may lead to lower bond strengths is the adhesive's low degree of conversion, which has been demonstrated for specific adhesive compositions [51].

Clearfil SE Bond (Kuraray) (Table 2), a two-step self-etch adhesive based on 10-methacryloyloxy decyl dihydrogen phosphate (10-MDP), is a reference for all other self-etch adhesives when it comes to dentin bond strengths [15,28]. In the author's laboratory, Clearfil S^3 Bond, the all-in-one successor of Clearfil SE Bond, shows lower dentin bond strengths than its predecessor. The pH of Clearfil S^3 Bond is less acidic than that of Clearfil SE Bond primer (2.4 versus 1.8, respectively). In spite of its relatively high pH, the bond strengths of Clearfil S^3 Bond on unground enamel are statistically similar to those of a more aggressive self-etch adhesive, Adper Prompt L-Pop (pH = 0.9–1.0) when tested in the author's laboratory. The manufacturer of Clearfil S^3 Bond claims that the difference between the two 10-MDP–based adhesives may lie on the "molecular dispersion technology" that keeps the homogeneity of Clearfil S^3 Bond adhesive and prevents phase separation that occurs with acetone-based all-in-one adhesives [21]. A recent study showed that Clearfil S^3 Bond is more resistant to mechanical stress than its two-bottle predecessor [52], which is surprising taking into consideration the excellent retention rates (above 90%) of Clearfil SE Bond in class-V clinical studies at 2 to 3 years [53,54]. This clinical behavior of both Clearfil adhesives denotes a good resistance to clinical fatigue of adhesives containing 10-MDP.

Table 2
Recent dentin adhesives

Adhesives and manufacturers		Composition	Instructions for use	Type
AdheSE	Ivoclar Vivadent	Primer: phosphoric acid acrylate, bis-acrylic acid amide, water, initiators, and stabilizers Bonding component: dimethacrylate, hydroxy ethyl methacrylate, highly dispersed silicon dioxide, initiators and stabilizers	1. Apply self-etch primer. Once the cavity is thoroughly coated, brush for 15s. Total reaction time should not be shorter than 30s. 2. Dry with mild airflow. 3. Apply self-etch bonding. 4. Dry with mild airflow. 5. Light cure for 10s.	Two-step self-etch
Adper Prompt L-Pop	3M ESPE	HEMA phosphates, HEMA, bis-GMA, modified polyalkenoic acid, water, photo-initiator	1. Activate the L-Pop Unit Dose Dispenser to mix the adhesive. 2. Apply mixed adhesive to entire surface, rubbing in the solution with moderate finger pressure for 15s. 3. Use a gentle stream of air to thoroughly dry the adhesive into a thin film. 4. Rewet the brush tip with adhesive and apply a second coat of adhesive to the tooth surface. The second coat does not require rubbing. 5. Use a gentle stream of air to thoroughly dry the adhesive into a thin film. 6. Light cure for 10s.	All-in-one self-etch, but requires mixing

Adper Single Bond Plus	3M ESPE	HEMA, bis-GMA, DMAs, methacrylate functional copolymer of polyacrylic and polyitaconic acids, water, ethanol, nanofiller, photo-initiator	1. Apply Scotchbond Etchant (35% silica-thickened phosphoric acid gel) to tooth surface for 15s. 2. Rinse thoroughly for 10s. 3. Blot excess water using a cotton pellet or mini-sponge. Do not air dry. 4. Apply 2–3 consecutive coats of adhesive for 15s with gentle agitation using a fully saturated applicator. 5. Gently air-thin for 5s to evaporate solvent. 6. Light cure for 10s.	Two-step etch and rinse
Clearfil S^3 Bond	Kuraray America	10-MDP, HEMA, bis-GMA, water, ethanol, silanated colloidal silica, camphorquinone	1. Thoroughly wet brush tip with Bond. Apply Bond to the tooth surface and leave in place for 20s. 2. Dry the entire surface sufficiently by blowing high-pressure air for more than 5s while spreading the bond layer thinly. 3. Light cure for 10s.	All-in-one self-etch

(continued on next page)

Table 2 (*continued*)

Adhesives and manufacturers	Composition	Instructions for use	Type
Clearfil SE Bond	Kuraray America	Primer: 10-MDP, HEMA, hydrophilic DMA, tertiary amine, water, photo-initiator Bonding: 10-MDP, HEMA, bis-GMA, hydrophilic DMA, tertiary amine, silanated colloidal silica, photo-initiator	1. Thoroughly wet brush tip with primer. Apply primer to the tooth surface and leave in place for 20s. 2. Dry with a mild air stream to evaporate the volatile ingredients. 3. Dispense the necessary amount of Bond into second mix well. 4. Apply Bond to the tooth surface. 5. After applying Bond, create a uniform film using a gentle air stream. 6. Light cure for 10s.	Two-step self-etch
G-Bond	GC America	4-MET, UDMA, phosphate monomer, DMA component, fumed silica filler, acetone, water, photo-initiator	1. Before dispensing, shake the bottle of G-Bond thoroughly. Replace bottle cap immediately after use. 2. Immediately apply to the prepared enamel and dentin surfaces using the microtip applicator. 3. Leave undisturbed for 10s. 4. After application, dry thoroughly using oil free air under maximum air pressure for 5s, in the presence of vacuum suction to prevent splatter of the adhesive. 5. Light cure 10s.	All-in-one self-etch

| iBond | Heraeus Kulzer | UDMA, 4-MET, glutaraldehyde, acetone, water, stabilizer, photo-initiator | 1. iBond is applied in three consecutive layers and massaged into the prepared hard-tooth structure for 30s.
2. Following that, the solution is blown away with a gentle air stream.
3. Polymerize for 20s. | All-in-one self-etch |
| Xeno IV | Dentsply Caulk | UDMA, PENTA, acetone, polymerizeable trimethacrylate resin, and two polymerizeable DMA resins, photo-initiator. | 1. Using the supplied disposable microbrush applicator tip, immediately apply and scrub surfaces with generous amounts of Xeno IV adhesive to thoroughly wet all the tooth surfaces for 15s.
2. Apply a second application of Xeno IV adhesive with the microbrush as above, scrubbing for 15s (20s for larger restorations).
3. Remove excess solvent by gently drying with clean, dry air from a dental syringe for at least 5s.
4. Cure Xeno IV adhesive for 10s. | All-in-one self-etch |

(continued on next page)

Table 2 (continued)

Adhesives and manufacturers		Composition	Instructions for use	Type
XP Bond	Dentsply DeTrey	Carboxylic acid modified dimethacrylate (TCB resin), PENTA, UDMA, TEGDMA, HEMA, butylated benzenediol (stabilizer), ethyl-4-dimethylaminobenzoate, camphorquinone, functionalized amorphous silica, t-butanol	1. Etch enamel for at least 15s and dentine for 15s or less with 36% phosphoric acid. 2. Wet all cavity surfaces uniformly with XP Bond in a disposable brush. Avoid pooling. 3. Leave the surface undisturbed for 20s. 4. Evaporate solvent by thoroughly blowing with air from an air syringe for at least 5s. The cavity surface should have a uniform, glossy appearance. Otherwise repeat steps 2 and 4. 5. Light-cure for a minimum of 10s. Ensure uniform exposure of all cavity surfaces. 6. Immediately place the restorative material over cured XP Bond.	Two-step etch and rinse

Abbreviations: bis-GMA, bisphenol glycidyl methacrylate; DMA, dimethacrylate; HEMA, 2-hydroxyethyl methacrylate; 10-MDP, 10-methacryloyloxy decyl dihydrogenphosphate; 4-MET, 4-methacryloxyethyl trimellitic acid; PENTA, dipentaerythritol penta-acrylate phosphate; TEGDMA, triethyleneglycol dimethacrylate; UDMA, urethane dimethacrylate.

Clinical performance of all-in-one adhesives

Some manufacturers of all-in-one self-etch adhesives do not recommend enamel pre-etching, while other manufacturers recommend phosphoric-acid etching of unground enamel. One would argue that additional enamel bond strength is always required to prevent marginal gaps and leakage. In a clinical setting, the adhesive is extended past the boundaries of the preparation, forming composite flashes. Bonding to this uninstrumented surface is needed to resist potential staining. The manufacturer of Xeno IV (Dentsply) recommends beveling the enamel margins for all procedures, which may be difficult to achieve in the cervical margin of class-II preparations. The manufacturers of Adper Prompt L-Pop (3M ESPE) and iBond (Heraeus Kulzer) do not recommend a separate enamel-etching step. The manufacturer of Clearfil S^3 Bond (Kuraray) recommends phosphoric-acid etching of unground enamel. Pre-etching may improve bonding to uninstrumented surfaces for all mild all-in-one adhesives, especially in areas where an adhesive flash formed during insertion. When enamel is etched separately, bond strengths increase significantly for self-etch adhesives [52,55]. However, if etching is extended to dentin, bonding may be compromised [52].

The enamel bond strengths of aggressive self-etch adhesives are usually higher than those of other self-etch adhesives [55], which may have to do with the relatively low pH compared with other less acidic adhesives (see Table 1). A recent morphological scanning electron microscopy study reported that the etching pattern on Adper Prompt, the bottle version of Adper Prompt L-Pop, is similar to that of phosphoric acid [56]. Other all-in-one adhesives, such as G-Bond (GC America) and iBond (Heraeus Kulzer), do not result in any discernible etching pattern or minimal exposure of crystallites in sporadic areas of unground enamel. On ground enamel, these adhesives result in islands of superficially dissolved enamel within areas without any sign of enamel dissolution (Fig. 15). One of the first clinical signs that a composite

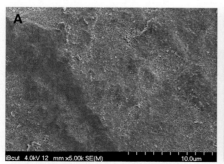 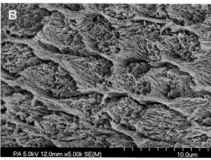

Fig. 15. (*A*) Field emission scanning electron micrograph of enamel treated with iBond (Heraeus Kulzer) after roughening the enamel with a diamond bur for 5 seconds. The adhesive was removed with acetone. (*B*) Enamel etched with 38% phosphoric acid (Pulpdent) for 15 seconds.

restoration is prone to failure is its early marginal staining. In fact, iBond is unable to penetrate the enamel smear layer [34], which explains why it is not very effective when applied on ground enamel. The almost inexistent etching pattern of iBond (an adhesive based on 4-methacryloxyethyl trimellitic acid (4-MET)) may have been responsible for massive marginal failure in a posterior composite clinical study at 1 year [57]. The all-in-one adhesive iBond resulted in statistically worse marginal staining than any of the other adhesives used in this study. Two other adhesives, a 10-MDP–based all-in-one adhesive (Clearfil S^3 Bond) and a self-etch adhesive based on polyalkenoic acid copolymer and hydroxyethyl-methacrylate (Adper Prompt L-Pop) resulted in a slightly lower percentage of excellent margins than the etch-and-rinse adhesive One-Step Plus, but these differences were not significant. At 1 year, the restorations inserted with iBond showed a dark orange aspect in most of the restorations, which was already evident at 6 months (Figs. 16 and 17). The change in color of the restoration might have been a result of the degradation of the adhesive itself, not that of the composite material, as the other adhesives did not result in such catastrophic results. This color change of the 4-MET–based all-in-one adhesive may be a result of its rapid hydrolysis, which is temperature-dependent and occurs as early as at 1 month, when specimens are stored at 25°C to 37°C [58].

Marginal adaptation is another parameter for which some self-etch adhesives result in unacceptable clinical results, which means they have a deficient enamel bonding ability. This bonding inability has been observed in laboratory studies as some all-in-one self-etch adhesives fail prematurely, with pretesting failures in the range of 50% [59]. Another study found 50% to 66% of pretesting failures with iBond with and without 20,000 cycles of thermal fatigue [33]. When the prevailing failure mode is adhesive, the bond strengths are generally low, while cohesive failures are more often associated with high bond strengths [60]. Several investigators have reported very low bond strengths with iBond when applied as per manufacturer's directions [37,61–63]. Clinically, iBond has resulted in more marginal staining than an etch-and-rinse adhesive in a class-V study [64], which corroborates the

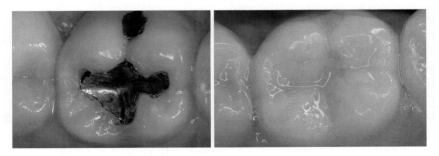

Fig. 16. Tooth #30 (*left*) preoperatively and (*right*) 1 year after being restored with the etch-and-rinse adhesive One-Step Plus (Bisco Inc.).

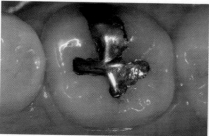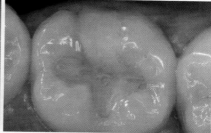

Fig. 17. Tooth #19 (*left*) preoperatively and (*right*) 1 year after being restored with the all-in-one self-etch adhesive iBond (Heraeus Kulzer) (same patient as in Fig. 15).

poor marginal staining observed in the 1-year posterior composite clinical study [57]. In that class-V study [64], iBond was compared with Gluma Solid Bond (Heraeus Kulzer), an etch-and-rinse adhesive, at 18 months. Other studies have also reported severe enamel microleakage in vitro, especially with thermal stresses with iBond [39,40], which explains the high percentage of marginal openings found clinically. Only 2 out of 27 iBond restorations were rated Alfa for marginal adaptation at 1 year [57].

According to the American Dental Association (ADA) guidelines for enamel and dentin adhesives, the cumulative incidence of clinical failures in each of two independent studies must be less than 10% to obtain full acceptance at 18 months [65]. While the enamel bonding ability of mild all-in-one adhesives may be jeopardized by thermal and mechanical fatigue, more aggressive all-in-one adhesives have resulted in acceptable clinical behavior [57,66]. At 18-months, 7% of the class-V restorations placed with Adper Prompt were lost versus none of the restorations inserted with Single Bond (3M ESPE), an etch-and-rinse adhesive [66]. The restorations bonded with Single Bond had slightly better marginal adaptation and marginal discoloration, but not statistically better. In spite of a slightly poorer clinical behavior at 18 months in class-V noncarious lesions, all-in-one adhesives like Adper Prompt have demonstrated lower bond strength to both enamel and dentin than one-bottle etch-and-rinse systems, such as Single-Bond [15,28,67].

In a posterior composite clinical study [57], marginal staining with Adper Prompt L-Pop at 1 year was not significantly different from baseline, but the P value was close to significance ($P = .06$). Marginal adaptation at 1 year was significantly worse than at baseline ($P < .0001$), as 18 out of 29 restorations were rated Bravo and 2 restorations were rated Charlie. Postoperative sensitivity to air at 1 year improved significantly for Adper Prompt L-Pop as compared with the preoperative values ($P < .016$). All 7 restorations that were sensitive to air preoperatively were not sensitive at 1 year.

While the aggressiveness (acidity) of the self-etch solution is important to determine the interaction depth of the restorative material with enamel, the chemical attributes of all-in-one adhesive are also important. Clinical studies with Prompt L-Pop, the predecessor of Adper Prompt, in cervical lesions resulted in a high failure rate [68,69]. The most crucial difference between the two versions is the presence of the polyalkenoic-acid copolymer in the latest versions (Adper Prompt and Adper Prompt L-Pop). This polyalkenoate-based component was first introduced in a resin-modified glass ionomer material (Vitrebond, 3M ESPE) and subsequently used in other formulations, including the adhesive systems (Scotchbond Multi-Purpose Primer and Single Bond). The polyalkenoate salt has been claimed to provide water stability to the adhesive system by a dynamic potential of breaking and renewing the bonding between the carboxyl groups and calcium, forming a stress-relaxation zone at the bonded interface [70].

Etch-and-rinse adhesives: Are they the benchmark for other adhesives?

Etch-and-rinse adhesives result in high enamel and dentin bond strengths. The enamel-etching pattern and the penetration into the dentinal substrate reinforce the idea that etch-and-rinse adhesives are still the benchmark for other adhesives when it comes to laboratory performance [26,27,47]. However, there are still concerns regarding the degree of infiltration of the etched dentin by some etch-and-rinse adhesives, such the ethanol- and water-based Single Bond, the unfilled version of Adper Single Bond Plus [71–73]. In spite of the high retention rate in clinical studies, reports have indicated that the bonds formed with Single Bond may undergo degradation in vivo at 1 year [73].

Acetone-based etch-and-rinse adhesives are more technique-sensitive than adhesives containing ethanol or water [74,75]. The clinical behavior of acetone-based etch-and-rinse adhesives may be determined by variations in the respective application technique, namely the amount of moisture left after rinsing the etchant and the amount of adhesive applied in the preparation [76]. One-Step Plus is the filled version of the acetone-based etch-and-rinse adhesive One-Step. Dentin bond strengths do not improve when the filled version is used [52,75]. Clinical studies using One-Step in class-V lesions have resulted in a wide variety of retention rates. One study found a retention rate of 75% at 3 years, while another study reported a 56% retention rate at 18 months [77,78]. Van Dijken [79] reported a 51% retention rate at 3 years, with higher failure rates in cervical lesions with sclerotic dentin. This low retention rate reported in some studies is not in agreement with the high dentin and enamel bond strengths found in other studies [80,81].

For multi-bottle etch-and-rinse adhesives, 5 full papers and 11 abstracts were published from 1998 to 2004 [82]. In 81% of the studies, multi-bottle etch-and-rinse adhesives fulfilled the full acceptance ADA guidelines (18 months), with an average annual failure rate of 4.8% [82]. With regard to one-bottle etch-and-rinse adhesives, 15 full papers and 17 abstracts appeared in the literature in the same period [82]. The clinical performance of multibottle etch-and-rinse adhesives was better than that of one-bottle etch-and-rinse adhesives, as only 51% fulfilled the full acceptance ADA guidelines (18 months) [81]. Even though dental adhesives have been available over several generations with an array of new materials being launched every year, clinical studies are not abundant in the literature. Several reasons may account for the discrepancy: first, the time constraints associated with setting up and running a clinical study with the respective periodic recalls; second, a generalized scarcity of industrial and independent funding for this type of applied research; and third, the frequent practice among manufacturers to launch a new version of a specific adhesive even before the previous one has been fully tested. As a result of all these limitations, researchers and clinicians still rely on data from laboratory studies to predict the behavior of adhesive materials.

Summary

Numerous simplified adhesives have been introduced to the dental market within the last few years, sometimes without comprehensive testing to validate the performance claimed by the respective manufacturers. Mild self-etch adhesives are unable to etch enamel to provide adequate retention for bonded restorations. Although high early resin–dentin bond strength values can be achieved with some self-etch adhesives, their resistance to thermal and mechanical stresses over time is disappointing. In light of the current drawbacks attributed to all-in-one self-etch adhesives, etch-and-rinse adhesives are still the benchmark for dental adhesion in routine clinical use.

Acknowledgments

The author gives special thanks to Drs. S. Duarte, G. Gomes, and M. Lopes for help preparing the scanning electron microscopy and transmission electron microscopy specimens.

References

[1] Buonocore MG. A simple method of increasing the adhesion of acrylic filling materials to enamel surfaces. J Dent Res 1955;34:849–53.
[2] Swift EJ, Perdigão J, Heymann HO. Bonding to enamel and dentin: a brief story and state of the art. Quintessence Int 1995;26:95–110.
[3] Baier RE. Principles of adhesion. Oper Dent Suppl 1992;5:1–9.
[4] Pashley DH. The effects of acid etching on the pulpodentin complex. Oper Dent 1992;17: 229–42.
[5] Asmussen E, Uno S. Adhesion of restorative resin to dentin: chemical and physicochemical aspects. Oper Dent Suppl 1992;5:68–74.
[6] Bowen RL, Eick JD, Henderson DA, et al. Smear layer: removal and bonding considerations. Oper Dent Suppl 1984;3:30–4.
[7] Eick JD, Cobb CM, Chapell RP, et al. The dentinal surface: its influence on dentinal adhesion. Part I. Quintessence Int 1991;22:967–77.

[8] Suzuki T, Finger WJ. Dentin adhesives: site of dentin vs. bonding of composite resins. Dent Mater 1988;4:379–83.

[9] Gwinnett AJ. Smear layer: morphological considerations. Oper Dent Suppl 1984;3:3–12.

[10] Perdigão J. Dentin bonding as function of dentin structure. Dent Clin North Am 2002;46: 1–25.

[11] Nakabayashi N, Kojima K, Masuhara E. The promotion of adhesion by the infiltration of monomers into tooth substrates. J Biomed Mater Res 1982;16:265–73.

[12] Brännström M, Nordenvall KJ. The effect of acid etching on enamel, dentin, and the inner surface of the resin restoration: a scanning electron microscopic investigation. J Dent Res 1977;56:917–23.

[13] Davidson CL, de Gee AJ, Feilzer A. The competition between the composite-dentin bond strength and the polymerization contraction stress. J Dent Res 1984;63:1396–9.

[14] Perdigão J, Lambrechts P, Van Meerbeek B, et al. The interaction of adhesive systems with human dentin. Am J Dent 1996;9:167–73.

[15] Van Meerbeek B, De Munck J, Yoshida Y, et al. Buonocore memorial lecture. Adhesion to enamel and dentin: current status and future challenges. Oper Dent 2003;28: 215–35.

[16] Pashley DH, Tay FR. Aggressiveness of contemporary self-etching adhesives. Part II: etching effects on unground enamel. Dent Mater 2001;17:430–44.

[17] Van Meerbeek B, Perdigao J, Lambrechts P, et al. The clinical performance of dentin adhesives. J Dent 1998;26:1–20.

[18] Tay FR, Pashley DH. Aggressiveness of contemporary self-etching systems. I: depth of penetration beyond smear layers. Dent Mater 2001;17:296–308.

[19] Perdigão J, Gomes G, Lopes MM. The influence of conditioning time on enamel adhesion. Quintessence Int 2006;37:41–7.

[20] Nishitani Y, Yoshiyama M, Wadgaonkar B, et al. Activation of gelatinolytic activity in dentin by self-etching adhesives. Eur J Oral Sci 2006;114:160–6.

[21] Van Landuyt KL, De Munck J, Snauwaert J, et al. Monomer-solvent phase separation in one-step self-etch adhesives. J Dent Res 2005;84:183–8.

[22] Carvalho RM, Stefano Chersoni S, Frankenberger R, et al. A challenge to the conventional wisdom that simultaneous etching and resin infiltration always occurs in self-etch adhesives. Biomaterials 2005;26:1035–42.

[23] Perdigão J, Geraldeli S. Bonding characteristics of self-etching adhesives to intact vs. prepared enamel. J Esthet Restor Dent 2003;15:32–42.

[24] Kanemura N, Sano H, Tagami J. Tensile bond strength to and SEM evaluation of ground and intact enamel surfaces. J Dent 1999;27:523–30.

[25] Van Meerbeek B, De Munck J, Mattar D, et al. Microtensile bond strength of an etch&rinse and self-etch adhesive to enamel and dentin as a function of surface treatment. Oper Dent 2003;28:647–60.

[26] Goracci C, Sadek FT, Monticelli F, et al. Microtensile bond strength of self-etching adhesives to enamel and dentin. J Adhes Dent 2004;6:313–8.

[27] Perdigão J, Gomes G, Duarte S Jr, et al. Enamel bond strengths of pairs of adhesives from the same manufacturer. Oper Dent 2005;30:492–9.

[28] Armstrong SR, Vargas MA, Fang Q, et al. Microtensile bond strength of a total-etch 3-step, total-etch 2-step, self-etch 2-step, and a self-etch 1-step dentin bonding system through 15-month water storage. J Adhes Dent 2003;5:47–56.

[29] Tay FR, Kwong S-M, Itthagarun A, et al. Bonding of a self-etching primer to non-carious cervical sclerotic dentin: interfacial ultrastructure and microtensile bond strength evaluation. J Adhes Dent 2000;2:9–28.

[30] De Munck J, Vargas M, Iracki J, et al. One-day bonding effectiveness of new self-etch adhesives to bur-cut enamel and dentin. Oper Dent 2005;30:39–49.

[31] Tay FR, Pashley DH, Suh BI, et al. Single-step adhesives are permeable membranes. J Dent 2002;30:371–82.

[32] Tay FR, Pashley DH. Water treeing—a potential mechanism for degradation of dentin adhesives. Am J Dent 2003;16:6–12.

[33] De Munck J, Van Landuyt K, Coutinho E, et al. Micro-tensile bond strength of adhesives bonded to class-I cavity-bottom dentin after thermo-cycling. Dent Mater 2005;21:999–1007.

[34] Frankenberger R, Tay FR. Self-etch vs etch-and-rinse adhesives: Effect of thermo-mechanical fatigue loading on marginal quality of bonded resin composite restorations. Dent Mater 2005;21:397–412.

[35] Bergenholtz G. Evidence for bacterial causation of adverse pulpal responses in resin-based restorations. Crit Rev Oral Biol Med 2000;11:467–80.

[36] Sensi LG, Lopes GC, Monteiro S Jr, et al. Dentin bond strength of self-etching primers/adhesives. Oper Dent 2005;30:63–8.

[37] Ito S, Tay F, Hashimoto M, et al. Effects of multiple coatings of two all-in-one adhesives on dentin bonding. J Adhes Dent 2005;7:133–41.

[38] Frankenberger R, Perdigao J, Rosa BT, et al. "No-bottle" vs "multi-bottle" dentin adhesives—a microtensile bond strength and morphological study. Dent Mater 2001;17:373–80.

[39] Brackett MG, Brackett WW, Haisch LD. Microleakage of Class V resin composites placed using self-etching resins: effect of prior enamel etching. Quintessence Int 2006;37:109–13.

[40] Kubo S, Yokota H, Yokota H, et al. Microleakage of cervical composites restored with one-step self-etch systems [abstract]. J Dent Res 2005;84(Spec Iss A).

[41] Pashley DH, Ciucchi B, Sano H, et al. Permeability of dentin to adhesive agents. Quintessence Int 1993;24:618–31.

[42] De Munck J, Van Meerbeek B, Yoshida Y, et al. Four-year water degradation of total-etch adhesives bonded to dentin. J Dent Res 2003;82:136–40.

[43] Hashimoto M, Tay FR, Ohno H, et al. SEM and TEM analysis of water degradation of human dentinal collagen. J Biomed Mater Res Part: B Appl Biomater 2003;66:289–98.

[44] Carrilho MR, Carvalho RM, Tay FR, et al. Durability of resin-dentin bonds related to water and oil storage. Am J Dent 2005;18:315–9.

[45] Hashimoto M, Ohno H, Sano H, et al. Micromorphological changes in resin-dentin bonds after 1 year of water storage. J Biomed Mater Res Part: B Appl Biomater 2002;63:306–11.

[46] Santerre JP, Shajii L, Leung BW. Relation of dental composite formulations to their degradation and the release of hydrolyzed polymeric-resin-derived products. Crit Rev Oral Biol Med 2001;12:136–51.

[47] Spreafico D, Semeraro S, Mezzanzanica D, et al. The effect of the air-blowing step on the technique sensitivity of four different adhesive systems. J Dent 2006;34:237–44.

[48] Tay FR, King NM, Chan KM, et al. How can nanoleakage occur in self-etching adhesive systems that demineralize and infiltrate simultaneously? J Adhes Dent 2002;4:255–69.

[49] Tay FR, Lai CN, Chersoni S, et al. Osmotic blistering in enamel bonded with one-step self-etch adhesives. J Dent Res 2004;83:290–5.

[50] Ito S, Hashimoto M, Wadgaonkar B, et al. Effects of resin hydrophilicity on water sorption and changes in modulus of elasticity. Biomaterials 2005;26:6449–59.

[51] Hoffmann M, Eppinger R, Kastrani A, et al. FTIR conversion analysis of all-in-one adhesives using different methods [abstract]. J Dent Res 2006;85(spec issue A).

[52] Can Say E, Nakajima M, Senawongse P, et al. Microtensile bond strength of a filled vs unfilled adhesive to dentin using self-etch and total-etch technique. J Dent 2006;34:283–91.

[53] Türkün SL. Clinical evaluation of a self-etching and an one bottle adhesive at two years. J Dent 2003;31:527–34.

[54] Van Meerbeek B, Kanumilli P, De Munck J, et al. A randomized controlled study evaluating the effectiveness of a two-step self-etch adhesive with and without selective phosphoric-acid etching of enamel. Dent Mater 2005;21:375–83.

[55] Miguez PA, Castro PS, Nunes MF, et al. Effect of acid-etching on the enamel bond of two self-etching systems. J Adhes Dent 2003;5:107–12.

[56] Di Hipolito V, de Goes MF, Carrilho MR, et al. SEM evaluation of contemporary self-etching primers applied to ground and unground enamel. J Adhes Dent 2005;7:203–11.

[57] Perdigão J, Dutra-Corrêa M, Castilhos N, et al. One-year clinical performance of self-etch adhesives in posterior restorations. Am J Dent, in press.
[58] Nishiyama N, Tay FR, Fujita K, et al. Hydrolysis of functional monomers in a single-bottle self-etching primer—correlation of ^{13}C NMR and TEM findings. J Dent Res 2006;85:422–6.
[59] Perdigão J, Gomes G, Gondo R, et al. In vitro bonding performance of all-in-one adhesives. Part I—microtensile bond strengths. J Adhes Dent 2006;8:367–73.
[60] Pereira PN, Okuda M, Sano H, et al. Effect of intrinsic wetness and regional difference on dentin bond strength. Dent Mater 1999;15:46–53.
[61] Atash R, Van den Abbeele A. Bond strengths of eight contemporary adhesives to enamel and to dentine: an in vitro study on bovine primary teeth. Int J Paediatr Dent 2005;15:264–73.
[62] Söderholm KJ, Guelmann M, Bimstein E. Shear bond strength of one 4th and two 7th generation bonding agents when used by operators with different bonding experience. J Adhes Dent 2005;7:57–64.
[63] Van Landuyt KL, Peumans M, De Munck J, et al. Extension of a one-step self-etch adhesive into a multi-step adhesive. Dent Mater 2006;22:533–44.
[64] Ritter AV, Heymann H, Pereira P, et al. Clinical evaluation of an all-in-one self-etching dental adhesive [abstract]. J Dent Res 2005;84(Spec Iss A).
[65] American Dental Association Council of Scientific Affairs. Acceptance program guidelines dentin and enamel adhesive materials. Available at: http://www.ada.org/ada/seal/standards/guide_materials_adhesive.pdf. Accessed February 10, 2007.
[66] Bittencourt DD, Ezecelevski IG, Reis A, et al. An 18-months' evaluation of self-etch and etch & rinse adhesive in non-carious cervical lesions. Acta Odontol Scand 2005;63:173–8.
[67] Inoue S, Vargas MA, Abe Y, et al. Microtensile bond strength of eleven contemporary adhesives to enamel. Am J Dent 2003;16:329–34.
[68] Brackett WW, Covey DA, St Germain HA Jr. One-year clinical performance of a self-etching adhesive in Class V resin composites cured by two methods. Oper Dent 2002;27:218–22.
[69] van Dijken JWV. Durability of three simplified adhesive systems in Class V non-carious cervical dentin lesions. Am J Dent 2004;17:27–32.
[70] Eliades GC. Dentine bonding systems. In: Vanherle G, Degrange M, Willems G, editors. State of the art on direct posterior filling materials and dentine bonding. Leuven (Belgium): Van der Poorten; 1993. p. 49–74.
[71] Wang Y, Spencer P, Hager C, et al. Comparison of interfacial characteristics of adhesive bonding to superficial versus deep dentine using SEM and staining techniques. J Dent 2006;34:26–34.
[72] Wang Y, Spencer P. Evaluation of the interface between one-bottle adhesive systems and dentin by Goldner's trichrome. Am J Dent 2005;18:66–72.
[73] Koshiro K, Inoue S, Tanaka T, et al. In vivo degradation of resin–dentin bonds produced by a self-etch vs. a total-etch adhesive system. Eur J Oral Sci 2004;112:368–75.
[74] Tay FR, Gwinnett JA, Wei SH. Micromorphological spectrum from overdrying to overwetting acid-conditioned dentin in water-free acetone-based, single-bottle primer/adhesives. Dent Mater 1996;12:236–44.
[75] Lee YK, Pinzon LM, O'Keefe KL, et al. Effect of filler addition on the bonding parameters of dentin bonding adhesives bonded to human dentin. Am J Dent 2006;19:23–7.
[76] Platt JA, Almeida J, Gozalez-Cabezas C, et al. The effect of double adhesive application on the shear bond strength to dentin of compomers using three one-bottle adhesive systems. Oper Dent 2001;26:313–7.
[77] Tyas MJ, Burrow MF. Three-year clinical evaluation of One-Step in non-carious cervical lesions. Am J Dent 2002;15:309–11.
[78] Brackett WW, Brackett MG, Dib A, et al. Eighteen-month clinical performance of a self-etching primer in unprepared class V resin restorations. Oper Dent 2005;30:424–9.
[79] Van Dijken JWV. Clinical evaluation of three adhesive systems in class V non-carious lesions. Dent Mater 2000;16:285–91.

[80] Loguerico AD, Uceda-Gomez N, Carrilho MR, et al. Influence of specimen size and regional variation on long-term resin-dentin bond strength. Dent Mater 2005;21:224–31.

[81] Reis A, Loguercio AD, Azevedo CL, et al. Moisture spectrum of demineralized dentin for adhesive systems with different solvent bases. J Adhes Dent 2003;5:183–92.

[82] Peumans M, Kanumilli P, De Munck J, et al. Clinical effectiveness of contemporary adhesives: a systematic review of current clinical trials. Dent Mater 2005;21:864–81.

THE DENTAL
CLINICS
OF NORTH AMERICA

ELSEVIER
SAUNDERS

Dent Clin N Am 51 (2007) 359–378

Aesthetic Anterior Composite Restorations: A Guide to Direct Placement

Brian P. LeSage, DDS[a,b,c,*]

[a]Beverly Hills Institute of Dental Esthetics, CA, USA
[b]UCLA Aesthetic Continuum, CA, USA
[c]Department of Restorative Dentistry, UCLA Dental School, CA, USA

Mastering anterior direct composite restorations is a necessity for the contemporary clinician who appreciates and understands the art and science of cosmetic dentistry. In the esthetic zone, composite bonding procedures are considered the most conservative and least invasive technique to return missing, diseased, and unsightly tooth structure to enhanced color, form, and function. The attractiveness and popularity of composites are easy to explain because these restorations have excellent esthetic potential, very good to excellent prognosis, and a reasonable fee [1,2].

Composites are the most versatile restorative material available to the dental professional, especially for the esthetic-conscious patients. The restorative dentist can use this versatile material in a mirage of indications and techniques. It is used as a direct and indirect restorative material on anterior and posterior teeth, orthodontics attachments and bracket cement, indirect restoration cements, correction of erosive and abfraction lesions, bases, liners, core build-ups and post and cores, mock-up for anterior esthetic or posterior occlusal trial therapy, splinting, provisionalization, gingival stabilization, and so forth.

For composite restorations to mimic natural tooth structure, the clinician must have a comprehensive understanding of the material science and techniques involved in direct bonding procedures. Material science can be broken down to include types of composites, tints, opaquers, adhesive systems, and armamentarium. The necessary techniques involve an understanding of color, adhesive principles, layering to create polychromicity, incisal effects and perfect imperfections, and finishing and polishing.

* 436 North Roxbury Drive, Suite 100, Beverly Hills, CA 90210.
   E-mail address: brian@cosmetic-dentistry.com

Composite materials

Composition

A composite is a multiphase substance formed from a combination of materials that differ in composition or form, remain bonded together, and retain their identities and properties [1]. They have four main components: (1) resin (organic polymer matrix); (2) filler (inorganic) particles; (3) coupling agent (silane); and (4) the initiator-accelerator of polymerization.

Resin matrix

Manufacturers prefer Bis-GMA resins because they have an aromatic structure that increases stiffness and compressive strength and lowers water absorption [2]. Bis-GMA 2,2-bis [4(2-hydroxy-3 methacryloyloxy-propyloxy)-phenyl] propane is the most popular dimethacrylate resin, but to accommodate better filler load triethylene glycol dimethacrylate or urethane dimethacrylate is added [3].

Fillers

Filler (inorganic) particles provide dimensional stability to the soft resin matrix [2]. The filler particles used in composites vary in size from less than 0.04 u to over 100 u. Common fillers are crystalline quartz; colloidal and pyrolytic silica; and such glasses as lithium, barium, or strontium silicate.

Coupling agent

Silane helps form a good bond between the resin matrix and filler particles during setting. The silane contains functional groups (eg, methoxy) that hydrolyze and react with the inorganic filler, and unsaturated organic groups that react with the resin matrix during polymerization [3].

Initiators and accelerators of polymerization

Composites contain initiators and accelerators that allow for light-, self-, and dual-cure modes. For visible light activation, camphoroquinones (0.03%–0.09%) start the free radical reaction using blue light in the 468 nm ± 20 nm range [2]. In the esthetic zone, light-cured composites are the material of choice because color matching and color stability are the most predictable.

For chemical-cured composites, aromatic tertiary amine (2%) initiates the free radical reaction when the paste and catalyst are mixed. Tertiary amines (and HEMA found in many adhesive systems) have been found to cause color change in composites on polymerization [4].

Classification and application

Historically, composites have been classified by particle size, shape, and distribution of fillers [5,6]. In the 1980s and 1990s, composite technology developed and became refined into two classifications: microhybrids and microfills. At the new millennium, nanotechnology introduced a new class of composite: the nanofillers. The three classifications of composites have their very distinct indications, advantages, and disadvantages (Table 1).

An ideal composite consists of the following four qualities: (1) mirror natural tooth structure in color and translucency; (2) strength to withstand function in stress-bearing areas for the long-term; (3) seamless or undetectable margins from restoration to tooth for the long-term; and (4) achieve the appropriate contour and polish (luster and finish) and maintain it for the long-term [7].

Microhybrid

Microhybrids contain a distribution of two or more irregular-shaped, but rather uniform diameter, "glass" or quartz particles of 0.2 to 3 μm plus 5% to 15% 0.04-μm microfine particles. This distribution of fillers makes the microhybrid 60% to 70% filled by volume, which translates roughly into 77% to 84% by weight [2,3,8] (Table 2).

The particle sizes and distribution and percent filled by weight lead to the following advantages for the microhybrid composite: strength; lower polymerization shrinkage (0.6%–1.4%); lower coefficient of thermal expansion; lower values of water sorption; higher flexural strength; and higher Knoop hardness [2,3,8]. Their disadvantage is maintaining a polish for the long-term.

Table 1
Indications, advantages, and disadvantages of the three major categories of composite resins

Classification	Indications	Advantages	Disadvantages
MicroHybrid	Layer the desired shade deep within the restoration to mimic dentin and enamel morphology Provide strength in any functional area	Strength: less likely to chip in high-strength area Refractory properties: opacity similar to enamel and dentin	Polishability: not long-term
MicroFill	Replace enamel in color and translucency Polish ability Wear resistance and surface texture	Polishability: high shine for the long-term Wear: resistance better than microhybrids Refractory properties: translucency similar to enamel	Lacks strength for some functional areas Can be too translucent
NanoFiller	All anterior and posterior restorative applications??	Potential advantages of MicroHybrid and MicroFill	No in vivo long-term studies

Table 2
Filler sizes in the three major categories of composite resins

Classification of composite	Size of filler particles (µm)	Volume of inorganic filler (%)	Filled by weight (%)	Diagram
MicroHybrid	0.2–3 plus 0.04	60–70	77–84	
MicroFill	0.02–0.04	32–50	50–70	
NanoFiller	0.01–0.04	60–72	79–84	

From an esthetic standpoint, microhybrids have more opacity and are excellent in replacing dentin. Microhybrids with smaller average particle sizes are excellent in replacing enamel and can be good to excellent in holding their polish over time. Examples of contemporary microhybrids include Herculite and Point 4 (Kerr/Sybron, Orange, California), Filtek Z250 (3M ESPE, St. Paul, Minnesota), and Vit~1~escence (Ultradent Products, Inc., South Jordan, Utah).

Microfills

Microfills contain colloidal silica fillers of 0.04-μm particle size and a filler loading of 32% to 50% by volume, which equates to 50% to 70% by weight [3,8] (see Table 2).

Because microfills are less highly filled, they have higher polymerization shrinkage, coefficient of thermal expansion, and water sorption compared with microhybrid composites. They demonstrate excellent polish and wear characteristics. Their disadvantage is strength and in some clinical situations being too translucent.

From an esthetic standpoint, microfills are superior to microhybrids. Microfills are excellent in replacing enamel, creating translucent zones, and having appropriate anatomy and high polish for the long-term. Examples of contemporary microfills include Filtek A110 (3M ESPE, St. Paul, Minnesota), Renamel (Cosmodent, Chicago, Illinois), and Matrixx Anterior Microfill (Discus Dental, Culver City, California).

Nanofillers

Two nanofillers are the aggregated zirconia-silica cluster filler (3M) with an average cluster particle size of 0.6 to 1.4 μm with primary particle size of 5 to 20 nm and a nonagglomerated-nonaggregated 20-nm silica filler [9]; and the Kerr prepolymerized filler (30–50 μm; barium glass, 0.4 μm; and silica nanoparticles, 0.02 μm). Nanofillers contain zirconia-silica nanocluster fillers of 30 to 50 μm (0.02 μm) plus submicron 0.01 to 0.02 μm silica particles. Nanofillers exhibit filler loading of 60% to 72% by volume, which equates to 79% to 84% by weight [9] (see Table 2). Examples of contemporary nanofillers include Premise (Kerr/Sybron, Orange, California), Aelite Aesthetic Enamel (Bisco, Schaumburg, Illinois), and Filtek Supreme Plus Universal Restorative (3M, St. Paul, Minnesota).

Being relatively new, nanofillers have few long-term in vivo studies, which is their disadvantage. Some shorter-term studies exist, and empirically this classification of composite has the potential to exhibit the advantages and limit the disadvantages of the other two composite classes. Because of their higher volume percent loading they exhibit lower shrinkage and associated less pull on margins, adhesives, and interproximal contact issues. More studies over a longer period of time are very much needed, however, to support such an opinion.

Adhesive systems and techniques

The success of composite restorations is directly related to the success of the adhesive system and technique used. Adhesive dentistry when applied correctly can prevent the dislodgement of composite restorations, prevent sensitivity issues, prevent microgap formation or microleakage leading to recurrent decay, and so forth. In article by Dr. Perdigao, a complete and comprehensive understanding of adhesives can be gained.

Tints

A tint is a color that is mixed with white. The tinted range of any one color can run from the pure color at its maximum intensity through to white [10]. For the restorative dentist, a tint's primary indication is to match natural tooth structure in polychromicity and maverick colors. It can also be used to help mask out the tooth-restoration interface. The effect on color is to lower the value. Tints are very intense colors and need to be used judiciously (Table 3).

Opaquers

Opacity is the opposite of transparency, and describes the degree to which light is prevented from passing through the color. It sometimes is described as "covering power," and is the color's ability to cover an underlying color, preventing any trace of the latter showing through [10].

The primary indication for an opaquer is to block out any size, shape, and degree of darkness within a tooth using only a thin layer of material. If the restorative dentist can create a stump shade that is uniform in polychromatic color, the final restoration need only reproduce the value and translucency of enamel. Opaquers can also help to block out the tooth-restorative interface and block out excessive translucency in CL III and IV restorations. Their effect on color is to raise value (see Table 3).

Table 3
Overview of tints and opaquers

	Indications
Tints	Match natural tooth structure in polychromicity and maverick colors
	Help mask out tooth-restorative interface
	Lower the value
Opaquers	Raise the value
	Block dark tooth color in thin layer
	Help mask out tooth-restorative interface
	Block excessive translucency in CL III and IV restorations

Layering techniques

Overview

When considering the direct anterior restoration in composite, one needs only to borrow from nature. If one studies and understands natural tooth structure in color, form, and function, then composite mirroring becomes the objective. Composite mirroring is the natural replacement of teeth with minimal or no additional removal of the intact, health dentition to normal form and function with tooth-colored material. With this approach, the restorative dentist must indulge the optical, anatomic, and functional characteristics of natural teeth.

In composite mirroring, the restorative dentist chooses an enamel and dentin replacement material that emulates the missing tooth structure in optical properties and strength. Clinically, this can be oversimplified by using a microhybrid in any area requiring strength or dentin replacement and a microfill for polishability and enamel replacement and effects (Fig. 1, Table 4). Figs. 2–5 shows a more in-depth breakdown of the composite mirroring system. Nanofillers, with more clinical data, may eventually eliminate the need for both systems.

When used properly, the composite mirroring system of layering is crucial in creating life-like restorations in strength and esthetics including polychromicity and incisal effects. The layering of composite material can be simple, involving one or two shades, or advanced, mimicking the artistic skills of the ceramic technician. When describing the four layering technique, trying to simplify or categorize which layering technique is

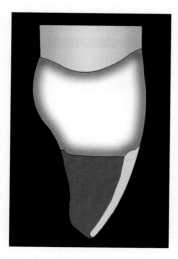

Fig. 1. Simplified, generalized overview of the composite mirroring system. Brown area using microhybrid for the stress-bearing zone (strength for the long-term), and beige area using a microfill for esthetics (polishability for the long-term). (*Courtesy of* Brian LeSage, DDS, Beverly Hills, CA.)

Table 4
Overview of tooth structure replacement and classification of composite resins

Tooth structure being replaced	Microhybrid	Microfill
Enamel: stress-bearing area	++++	+ (need support of tooth)
Enamel: pure esthetic area	++~+++	++++
Dentin: pure esthetic area (ie, CL III, V)	+++~++++	+++~++++ (higher chroma needed)
Dentin: stress-bearing area (ie, CL IV)	++++	+ (need support of MicroHybrid)

Abbreviations: ~, not indicated; +, least indicated; ++++, highly indicated.

best, the clinician needs to consider the patient's financial commitment and the esthetic wants of the patient. Visualization, being able to see and believe in creating the end point, is critical. The purpose of composite layering is to establish the dentin layer and dentinal lobes in a tooth and create the wonderful nuances of enamel and enamel effects that transform into incisal translucency and incisal halo effects [7,11–16,17–21].

Shade selection technique

The shade selection technique is as follows [18,22–26]:

1. Pumice tooth lightly to remove any stains, debris, pellicle, and so forth, but not so much as to influence the tooth's natural luster and finish. Otherwise, this could affect the predictability of shade matching (Fig. 6A).
2. The dentin shade is best obtained from the gingival third of the tooth where the enamel is the thinnest (Fig. 6B) or from the canines where

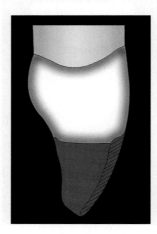

Fig. 2. Simple layering technique. Brown area demonstrating the use of one shaded material, and the hashed zone an optional second shaded material of different opacities and the same or different chroma range. (*Courtesy of* Brian LeSage, DDS, Beverly Hills, CA.)

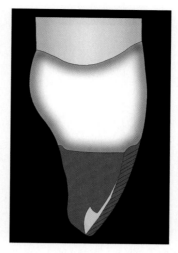

Fig. 3. Less simple layering technique. Same as simple layering technique with the addition of a translucent zone internally to help distinguish the dentinal lobes and create incisal effects. (*Courtesy of* Brian LeSage, DDS, Beverly Hills, CA.)

the chroma is the greatest. Clinically, this is done by placing a small thin convenience form of the anticipated shade in the gingival third and light curing. This must be done before the teeth dehydrate. It should be noted that microhybrids generally get darker on light curing, and microfills get lighter when light cured.

3. The enamel shade is conveniently obtained in the middle third of the tooth, where the enamel is the thickest (Fig. 6C).

4. The incisal or translucent shade is observed in the incisal third of the tooth, where the enamel is the thickest and there is little dentin opacity. In most anterior teeth the translucent zone is not limited to the incisal edge but carries into the transitional line angle zones (Fig. 6D).

5. Color mapping by the clinician doing the esthetic composite restoration aids the clinician because these procedures can be lengthy and often the operator's eyes fatigue physically and mentally. The color map is a picture or prescription to be used as a guide throughout the fabrication of the direct restoration (Fig. 6E).

6. Practice mock-up using the selected shades can be done quickly without good adhesive technique to act as a shade evaluation guide and subsequently to fabricate a putty matrix. Once one is satisfied with the color based on the mock-up, the clinician turns their attention to contour. Modify the mock-up to obtain the correct outline form, embrasure form, incisal edge, and incisal plane contour to the facial-incisal line angle (do not spend time getting the facial surface ideal at this point). At the same time, get the centric stops and anterior disclusion that is needed for longevity. Once the occlusion and contours

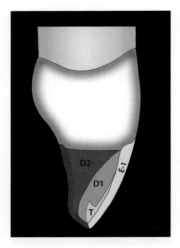

Fig. 4. 3-D Advanced Layering Technique. Brown area demonstrating the use of TWO opacious shaded materials varying in chroma (D2-Higher Chroma Dentin opacious shade, D1-Lower Chroma Dentin opacious shade) and a translucent zone (T) internally to help distinguish the dentinal lobes and additionally an outer layer of enamel material (E) of the same or different chroma range. Lingual hashed enamel layer can be the E shade or the D2 shade. (*Courtesy of* Brian LeSage, DDS, Beverly Hills, CA.)

are correct, use a stiff VPS material, such as Aquasil Ultra Rigid (Dentsply/Caulk), Affinity (Clinician's Choice), Imprint II (3M ESPE), and Exaimplant (GC), to fabricate a putty matrix that captures the entire lingual contour completely to the facial-incisal line angle [27] (Fig. 6F, G, and H).

Simple layering technique

This technique should be considered for the patient who has minimal esthetic concerns, but when all decisions are based on economics. One or two shaded materials (with different opacities and the same or different chroma range) suffice (see Fig. 2).

Less simple layering technique

This technique should be considered for the patient who has moderate esthetic concerns, but when decisions are based primarily on economics. It entails one or two shaded materials (with different opacities and the same or different chroma range) and another layer using incisal shaded material (Fig. 3).

Three-dimensional advanced layering technique

This technique should be considered for the patient who has a moderate to extensive understanding of esthetics and when finances play minimally

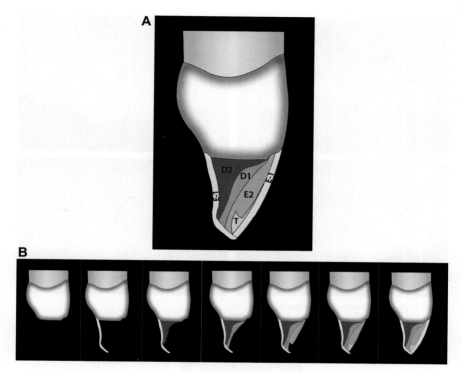

Fig. 5. (*A*) 3-D Characterized Layering Technique. Same as 3-D Advanced Layering technique with the lingual enamel layer being a distinct (E) layer. And the addition of a second facial enamel layer of differing chroma range to internally give depth to the dentinal lobes and create incisal effects mirroring mother nature. Not shown is the tint layer placed internally creating maverick colors and effects. (*B*) Sequential application and layering starting from the lingual and extending to the facial with multiple dentin and enamel shades, and a translucent shade. (*Courtesy of* Brian LeSage, DDS, Beverly Hills, CA.)

into their decision-making process. Two shaded materials with different chromas are used to replace dentin, with an enamel layer for enamel effects and another layer using incisal shaded material (Fig. 4).

Three-dimensional characterized layering techniques

This technique should be considered for the patient who has a very high esthetic intelligence quotient and is very esthetically demanding, and when finances are not part of their decision-making process. Two shaded materials with different chromas are used to replace dentin, two shaded materials with different chromas are used for the enamel layer for enamel effects, and another layer uses incisal shaded material. A characterization layer is placed between the incisal and enamel layers or the two enamel layers depending on the intensity of the effect desired (Fig. 5). Tints are placed internally to

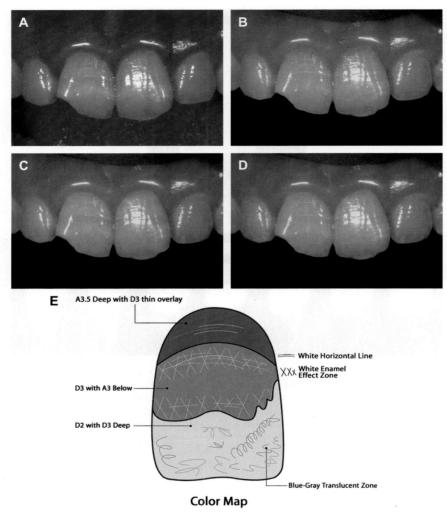

Color Map

Fig. 6. Shade Selection Technique. (*A*) Before picture at 1:1 showing worn and chipped areas after lightly pumicing. (*B*) Highlighted gingival 1/3 for dentin shade selection. (*C*) Highlighted middle 1/3 for enamel shade selection. (*D*) Highlighted incisal 1/3 for translucent shade selection. (*E*) Color mapping to aid in shade predictability. (*F*) Mock-up used for preliminary shade determination and 3-D spatial relations to fabricate putty matrix. (*G*) Putty Matrix trimmed properly to the facial incisal line angle. Note bevel and star burst bevel. (*H*) Final restoration appearing seamless and mirroring mother nature. (*Courtesy of* Brian LeSage, DDS, Beverly Hills, CA.)

mirror the unique characterizations of the natural tooth, such as subsurface staining or demarcations of any color, shape, or size.

The outer layer is unique and preplanned in this technique. If the desired outcome is a brighter (higher value) shaded tooth, then the outer layer must have enamel color. Enamel shade should be used a the outer layer and the

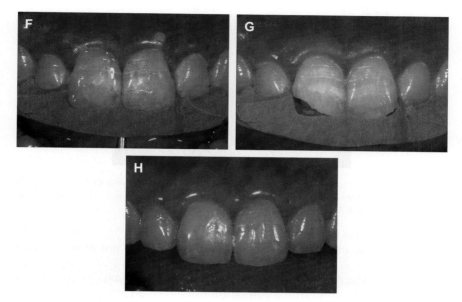

Fig. 6 (*continued*)

incisal shade internally. If the final outcome desired is a tooth with lower value, then the outer layer is the translucent shade, which on top of the last enamel shade acts as a transparent filtering layer resulting in a lower value.

As the complexity of the layering technique occurs, it is important to evaluate each layer from the incisal view and sagittal view. The clinician needs to be aware if they are in the dentin substitute zone or enamel substitute zone. If the various layers are added too thick, all additional layers are too far facial and removed in the contour and finishing phase.

Seamless margins

The purpose of composite layering is to establish the dentin layer and dentinal lobes in a tooth and create the wonderful nuances of enamel and enamel effects that transform into incisal translucency and incisal halo effects. If these layers have voids or are not seamless, breakdown of the restoration or the tooth restoration interface is detected early. Listed are multiple steps that must be followed to created undetectable margins [7,20,28,29]:

1. Place a proper bevel.
    a. Facially on enamel: 2-mm knife-edge type. An additional starburst bevel with varying depths and lengths is an added benefit. These multiple bevels extend from the cavosurface margin outward, some remaining only in enamel and others depths involving dentin (Fig. 7).

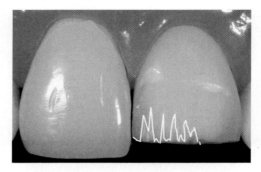

Fig. 7. Typical 2 mm long knife-edge bevel from mesial to distal; white line shows variability in depth and length of starburst design on mesial half of incisal edge. (*Courtesy of* Brian LeSage, DDS, Beverly Hills, CA.)

    b. Facially on dentin: no bevel, butt margin.

    c. Lingually on enamel: chamfer margin preferably not in the contact zone.

2. Etch past the end of the bevel. By etching past the enamel bevel, the clinician is able to finish the composite to infinity slightly past the end of the bevel. This technique makes for a disappearing margin and allows for further longevity of the restoration because future polishing becomes necessary in the maintenance phase.

3. Roll the outer layer with clean gloved hands for sculptability and to prevent inclusions or voids. Once the convenience form of the desired shade of material is removed from the composite container, it has a cut or white chalky nature to the edge. If used right out of the container this zone may show up as a void in the final restoration. By taking the allocated amount of material and rolling it in clean gloved hands one can accomplish two important roles: the material is warmed slightly and is now in a better sculptable state, and the cut portion is not detectable because it is one uniform mass.

4. Sculpt the outer layer and get the geometric outline form, transition line angles, and primary anatomy to approximately 85% before curing. This can involve leaving the interproximal matrix (Mylar plastic strips; Composi-Tight metal matrix, Garrison Dental Solutions; Palodent metal matrix, Dentsply/Caulk) in place or removing it by pulling toward the lingual and using composite instruments and brushes to contour before light curing.

5. Super cure the composite and wait 10 minutes before finishing. Because composites cannot be overcured and the conversion is never 100%, it is best to super cure to maximize the physical properties of the material. The material continues to cure even after the light is removed; give the material time to relax before finishing.

6. Finish the margin back to between the etch and the end of the bevel. As described in step 1, the composite should be finished out to infinity. By

ending this margin slightly past the bevel, as the margins pick up stain over time there is a very thin zone of material that still remains polishable and easy to maintain.

7. Rotate finishing armamentarium from restoration to tooth. When using rubber or silicone finishing discs embedded with silicon carbide, aluminum oxide (degrees of grit) to prevent the grit from embedding in the margin, have the disc spinning from restoration to tooth.

8. Do not use rubber on the margins. Many manufacturers have excellent rubber polishing systems. These are best used in the body of the restoration and not at the margins because the rubber shavings can get embedded in the margin.

9. High polish appropriate for the natural dentition. An appropriate polish and luster is the key that maintains itself for the long-term (see section on polish and finishing).

Customization

Overview

In the composite mirroring layering technique, the ultimate result was obtained by using four to five different shaded or translucent materials with a very particular objective in mind. Tints were also mentioned, but the technique or application is now described.

There are five easily learned techniques to mirror the natural dentition in check lines, spots, craze lines, and any other maverick color issues seen in nature. It must be noted that tints are very strong, and while performing the layering technique many times the tints tend to disappear. They reappear as the polishing sequence progresses. Tints must never be placed on the surface, because finishing and polishing lead to their removal. Tints can be mixed to create a unique, desired color. The five techniques to creating a natural craze line are as follows:

1. Paint and thin: Using a thin paintbrush with the desired tint, usually white or brown, place the tint to mirror the adjacent tooth. The tint is on the tooth but way too wide and so thin the material from both sides leaves a thin, nonstraight line. Then light cure.

2. Scar and paint: Scar or scribe the tooth with a thin metal disc (VisionFlex, Brasseler, Savannah, Georgia) or diamond bur. Paint the desired colored tint in the scribed area and clean the excess. Then light cure (Fig. 8).

3. Matrix: After placing the second-to-most outer layer and before curing, place a Mylar or metal matrix into the composite, preferably nonstraight, and light cure. Remove the matrix, paint the desired colored tint in the grooved area, and clean the excess. Then light cure.

4. Vertical wall for depth: While placing the second-to-most outer layer create a wall in the composite, preferably nonstraight, and light cure.

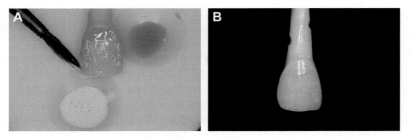

Fig. 8. (*A*) Tint application internally showing lines and dot maverick colors in second-to-last layer. (*B*) The final restoration. (*Courtesy of* Brian LeSage, DDS, Beverly Hills, CA.)

Paint the desired colored tint on the walled area and clean the excess. Then light cure.

5. Anneal material over the tint: While placing the most outer enamel or dentin layer create a notch or groove in the composite, preferably non-straight. Paint the desired colored tint in the notched or grooved area and anneal the composite toward and within itself, preferably in a non-straight pattern. Then light cure.

These techniques are best to learn on extracted teeth or typodont teeth, where the skills can be perfected in a nonclinical setting. Habituation is needed to master any new technique.

Finishing and polishing

This is considered by many to be the most difficult phase of anterior composite restorations. If the clinician follows the described guidelines of this article, this step becomes routine and not one to be feared. Finishing and polishing is crucial in finalizing the composite restoration to mimic nature in form, function, and longevity [30].

There is no shortcut in fabricating life-like restorations. Properly finished and polished composites allow for a proper seal of the restoration, which influences its durability and allows for minimal stain accumulation, less plaque accumulation, and better wear resistance and marginal integrity [28,29,31,32]. The finishing sequence includes diamond burs, followed by polishing discs or rubber polishing discs, points, wheels, and polishing with buffing wheels and polishing paste.

Diamonds burs, specifically submicron diamonds of 50 μm or less UCLA LeSage Anterior Preparation Bur System (Brasseler USA, Savannah, Georgia), run with copious amounts of water are used to create and modify the restoration to the proper geometric outline form and contours, including the proper line angles and primary and some secondary anatomy [33]. As seen in Fig. 9, blue articulating paper can help guide the clinician through this process. In conjunction, course and fine polishing disc (KerrHawe, Kerr,

Orange, CA; EP Polishers, Brasseler, Savannah, GA; Sof-Flex Disc, 3M, St. Paul, MN; Flexi-discs, Cosmodent, Chicago, IL) run with copious amounts of water can be used to get to hard-to-reach areas to refine the aforementioned anatomic landmarks. Many times the loss of secondary anatomy is seen after this step. With the aid of electric handpieces (Ti-Max NL 400, NSK, Brasseler, Savannah, Georgia) and diamond burs, the clinician can re-establish the primary and secondary anatomy. One should check for stable centric stops and appropriate anterior disclusion. The finishing phase is not complete until interproximally and gingivally no overhangs remain and the geometric outline form is complete.

Gingivally, the use of hand instrumentation may be more ideal to remove flashing or potential overhanging material. Bard-Parker #12 or #15 blades are probably most popular, but carbide composite carvers are considered equally effective. The carbide carvers (Brasseler, Savannah, Georgia) come in several shapes matching closely to the gingival area of intended use.

Interproximally, the use of metal finishing strip (VisionFlex Strips, Brasseler, Savannah, GA, GC International Metal Strips, GC America, Alsip, IL) will initiate the bulk reduction. To make appropriate embrasures, the use of an interproximal diamond disc is needed. Embrasures need to be defined by depth and volume, and the best way to accomplish this is with thin diamond discs (VisionFlex Disc, Brasseler, Savannah, Georgia) on a straight or contra-angle. Completing the finishing and polishing of the interproximal and transition zones is crucial, because these areas are more prone to stain and plaque accumulation. The use of plastic interproximal strips (Sof-Lex Strips, 3M, St. Paul, MN; Vivadent Strips, Vident, Brea, CA) of two grits is essential to attain the ideal polished surface in this stain-susceptible zone.

Texture creation is the tertiary anatomy that makes an average composite restoration become life-like. Several possible techniques to consider are

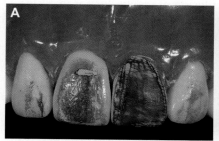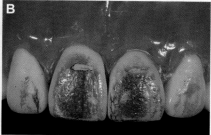

Fig. 9. Technique showing the use of articulating paper to mirror primary and secondary anatomy. (*A*) Once primary anatomy is close, smudge articulating paper across entire surface of tooth; note flatness and no facial anatomy or texture in facial veneer restoration on tooth #9. (*B*) Articulating paper confirming primary, secondary, and tertiary anatomy in direct composite restoration mirroring that of adjacent tooth #8. (*Courtesy of* Brian LeSage, DDS, Beverly Hills, CA.)

tapping or dragging a course or medium diamond bur or disc with an air or electric handpiece, using the corner or side of a cross-cut fissure bur, or using a white or green stone with various motions. This completes the finishing phase. All that is left is to establish the appropriate polish and luster.

To obtain the appropriate high polish the use of chammy-type buffing wheels and discs (Flex-Buff Disc, Cosmedent; Chammy wheel, Brasseler, Savannah, Georgia) on contra-angle and straight slow-speed handpiece is required. The use of a polishing paste (Luster Paste, Kerr, Orange, CA; Enamelize, Cosmodent, Chicago, IL; Truluster, Brasseler, Savannah, GA; or Prisma-Gloss, Dentsply/Caulk, Milford, DE) wet then dry will add gloss to the final restoration.

Created is a composite restoration that not only mimics the beauty of dentin and enamel, but also defies detection. There are still two remaining steps to consider. The first is to clean, etch, rinse, and place a seal or glaze (BisCover LV, Bisco) on the restoration to seal any microcracks or microsurface defects from staining. The second is to take photos for self-evaluation and return of the patient with in 5 days (prescheduled) to make any alterations detected in the photography and modify any occlusal contacts, especially in anterior guidance movements.

Summary

Taking a systematic approach to direct composite restorations can greatly enhance the outcome of this multifaceted discipline. To enjoy the true art and science of cosmetic dentistry, the clinician must have a thorough understanding of tooth morphology and topography; tooth shade analysis; composite systems and layering techniques; and the use of tints, opaquers, and maverick colors and zones to create restorations that mimic nature. Once the diseased, missing, or unsightly tooth structure has the exquisite beauty of enamel and dentin in depth of color, contour, and light reflection, the finishing and polishing creates the illusion of reality. Factor in occlusion and maintenance, and direct composite restorations are the most unique and conservative restorations mirroring the reality of a tooth.

References

[1] Lee SM. Preface. Dictionary of composite materials technology. Lancaster (PA): Techmic Publishing Company; 1989.
[2] Albers HF. Tooth colored restorations: principles and techniques. 9th edition. BC Decker Publishing; 2002.
[3] Craig R, Powers J. Restorative dental materials. Chapter 9. 11th edition. Mosby; 2002.
[4] Suh B. Update on adhesive dentistry. Presented at International Adhesive Symposium. Schaumburg (IL): Bisco, February 2007.
[5] Terry D. Application of nanotechnology. Editorial Commentary, Pract Periodontics Aesthet Dent 2004;16(3):220–2.

[6] Leinfelder KF, Sluder TB, Sockwell CL, et al. Clinical evaluation of composite resins as anterior and posterior restorative materials. J Prosthet Dent 1975;33(4):407–16.
[7] Eubank J, LeSage B. Presented at the UCLA aesthetic continuum, composite lecture and hands-on workshops, 1997–2006. UCLA Dental School, Los Angeles.
[8] O'Brien WJ, editor. Dental materials and their selection. 3rd edition. Carol Stream (IL): Quintessence Publishing Co; 2002. p. 114–6.
[9] Mitra S, Wu D, Holmes B. An application of nanotechnology in advanced dental material. J Am Dent Assoc 2003;134(10):1382–90.
[10] Sidaway I. Color mixing bible. NY: Watson-Guptill Publication; 2002.
[11] Dietschi D. Free-hand composite resin restorations: a key to anterior aesthetics. Pract Periodontics Aesthet Dent 1995;7(7):15–27.
[12] Dietschi D, Dietschi JM. Current developments in composite materials and techniques. Pract Periodontics Aesthet Dent 1996;8:603–14.
[13] Dietschi D. Free-hand bonding in the esthetic treatment of anterior teeth: creating the illusion. J Esthet Dent 1997;9(4):156–64.
[14] Dietschi D, Ardu S, Krejci I. Exploring the layering concepts for anterior teeth. In: Rouley JF, Degrange M, editors. Adhesion: the silent revolution in dentistry. Chicago: Quintessence; 2000. p. 235–51.
[15] Chiche G, Pinault A. Aesthetic of anterior fixed prosthodontics. Chicago: Quintessence; 1994.
[16] Dietschi D. Layering concepts in anterior composite restorations. J Adhes Dent 2001;3: 71–80.
[17] Gordon AA, vonderLehr WN, Herrin HK. Bond strength of composite to composite and bond strength of composite to glass ionomer lining cements. Gen Dent 1986;34: 290–3.
[18] Terry D, Leinfelder K. An integration of composite resin with natural tooth structure: the CL IV restoration. Pract Proced Aesthet Dent 2004;16(3):235–42.
[19] Miller M. Reality: the information source for esthetic dentistry. Houston (TX): Reality Publishing; 2006.
[20] Fahl NJ. Predictable aesthetic reconstruction of fractured anterior teeth with composite resins: a case report. Pract Periodontics Aesthet Dent 1996;8(1):17–30.
[21] Devoto W. Clinical procedure for producing aesthetic stratified composite resin restorations. Pract Proced Aesthet Dent 2002;14(7):541–3.
[22] Sproul RC. Color matching in dentistry. Part 1. The three-dimensional nature of color. J Prosthet Dent 2001;86:453–7.
[23] Hall NR, Kafalias MC. Composite colour matching: the development and evaluation of a restorative colour matching system. Aust Prosthodont J 1991;5:47–52.
[24] Vanini L. Light and color in anterior composite restorations. Pract Periodontics Aesthet Dent 1996;8(7):673–82.
[25] Deliperi S, Bardwell DN, Congiu MD. Reconstruction of severely damaged endodontically treated and bleached teeth using a microhybrid composite resin: two-year case report. Pract Proced Aesthet Dent 2003;15(3):221–6.
[26] Vanini L, Mangani FM. Determination and communication of color using the five color dimensions of teeth. Pract Proced Aesthet Dent 2001;13(1):19–26.
[27] Behle C. Placement of direct composite veneers utilizing a silicone build-up guide and intraoral mock-up. Pract Periodontics Aesthet Dent 2001;12(3):259–66.
[28] Jefferies SR, Barkmeier WW, Gwinnett AJ. Three composite finishing systems: a multisite in vitro evaluation. J Esthet Dent 1992;4(6):181–5.
[29] Goldstein RE. Finishing of composite and laminates. Dent Clin North Am 1999;33(2): 305–18.
[30] Miller M. Contouring and polishing resin-based materials. Reality; the techniques. 2003;1:23–29.

[31] Powers JM, Fan PL, Raptis CN. Color stability of new composite restorative materials under accelerated aging. J Dent Res 1980;59(12):2071–4.

[32] Sarac D, Sarac SY, Kulunk S. The effects of polishing techniques on the surface roughness and color change of composite resins. J Prosthet Dent 2006;96:33–40.

[33] Blitz N. Diagnosis and treatment evaluation in cosmetic dentistry: a guide to accreditation criteria. American Academy of Cosmetic Dentistry; Madison (WI).

ELSEVIER
SAUNDERS

Dent Clin N Am 51 (2007) 379–397

THE DENTAL
CLINICS
OF NORTH AMERICA

Abrasive Finishing and Polishing in Restorative Dentistry: A State-of-the-Art Review

Steven R. Jefferies, MS, DDS

*Department of Restorative Dentistry, Temple University School of Dentistry,
3223 North Broad Street, Philadelphia, PA 19140, USA*

Effective finishing and polishing of dental restorations not only result in optimal aesthetics but also provide for acceptable oral health of soft tissues and marginal integrity of the restorative interface. In an earlier published review article, this author noted some of the difficulties resulting from improperly finished and polished restorations, including "excessive plaque accumulation, gingival irritation, increased surface staining, and poor or suboptimal esthetics of the restored teeth" [1]. This review of abrasive technology in dentistry provides an overview of basic principles of abrasive science and considers some research concerning clinically relevant questions involving this subject. The article also discusses some recent innovations in finishing and polishing devices in restorative dentistry. This review brings forward some newly published, outcome-based information concerning the relevance and importance of an effective knowledge of finishing and polishing techniques and materials. The overall aim is to provide the reader with an enhanced awareness and broader knowledge of the principles and tools available to produce optimal surface finishing and integrity in dental restoratives.

Basic principles of tribiology as it relates to abrasive science in dentistry

The mechanisms involved in mechanical finishing and polishing using abrasive particles are part of tribology, the discipline associated with material science, physics, chemistry and surface-contact engineering [2]. A description of a tribiological system consists of a set of experimental

E-mail address: steven.jefferies@temple.edu

0011-8532/07/$ - see front matter © 2007 Elsevier Inc. All rights reserved.
doi:10.1016/j.cden.2006.12.002

dental.theclinics.com

parameters (eg, applied load, velocity, and duration of motion) and the system structure (eg, the two bodies in contact, the interfacial media, and the surrounding media).

Finishing and polishing devices, materials, and procedures are intended to produce intentional, selective, and controlled wear of dental restorative-material surfaces. Wear is defined as a cumulative surface damage phenomenon in which material is removed from a body as small debris particles, primarily by mechanical processes. The wear mechanism is the transfer of energy with removal or displacement of material. The four major wear mechanisms are adhesion, abrasion, surface fatigue, and tribochemical reactions. In polishing with abrasive particles, the wear mechanism is mostly abrasive wear, but other mechanisms are also possible. These include surface fatigue and the development of ploughing grooves or scratches, which in some instances are accompanied by hertzian fractures. For the classification of the abrasive-wear modes, this article uses the most widely accepted terms. These are two-body abrasion and three-body abrasion. These terms illustrate the experimental situations encountered in finishing and polishing techniques, as illustrated in Fig. 1. In a two-body mode, the bound abrasive particle is solidly fixed to the substrate (see Fig. 1). In a three-body abrasive mode, free (or loose) particles form slurry between the specimen surface to be polished and a flat polishing substrate (see Fig. 1). The free particles in a three-body wear mode may be intentionally added abrasives or detached debris from the worn surface. Most dental finishing and polishing devices operate in the two-body mode. Nevertheless, dentist, hygienists, and laboratory technicians use the three-body abrasive mode in the form of loose abrasives, such as prophy or polishing pastes.

Three-body abrasive wear occurs when loose particles move in the interface between the specimen surface and the polishing application device. Such a situation occurs when abrasives are intentionally deposited so as to roll on top of the polishing substrate, as in the case of the final polishing

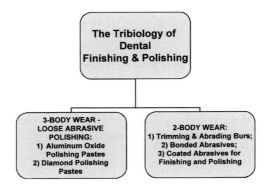

Fig. 1. Finishing and polishing procedures in restorative dentistry follow tribiologic principles of abrasive wear in two-body and three-body configurations.

step with very small grains on soft lubricated pads. A three-body mode may also occur when small pieces of material are detached from the specimen to be polished and become trapped or circulate within the zone of contact between the two first bodies.

The manifestations of abrasive wear are a change of the surface roughness resulting from material removal and a change of the physical and chemical properties of the surface and subsurface with respect to those of the bulk. These deformations, which can be described in mechanical and geometrical terms, are accompanied by the production of highly localized heat and the creation of residual defects and surface flaws in the material being polished.

Why the interest in finishing and polishing in dentistry?

Dentists have always been encouraged to take the time and effort to adequately finish and polish restorations. The clinical and scientific reasons for careful finishing and polishing have been noted [3]:

1. To remove excess flash and refine the margins of the restoration
2. To reduced the risk of fracture, since a rough surface may be more likely to fracture
3. To reduce surface imperfections, hence reducing surface area and thus reducing the risk of surface breakdown and corrosion
4. To produce a smooth surface less likely to retain plaque
5. To improve oral function and mastication, since food slides more easily over polished tooth surfaces
6. To produce smooth surfaces that facilitate oral hygiene procedures with access to all surfaces, marginal areas, and interproximal areas through normal toothbrushing and use of dental floss
7. To produce smooth restoration contacts, leading to less wear on opposing and adjacent teeth
8. To produce a more aesthetic, light-reflectant restoration for the patient

This article later reviews in greater depth some of the literature-based evidence regarding these clinical issues.

Just what do we mean by finishing and polishing?

Finishing and polishing refers to gross contouring of the restoration, to obtain the desired anatomy, and the reduction and smoothing of the roughness and scratches created by finishing instruments. The terms, definitions, and procedural steps involved in the finishing and polishing underscore some confusion about the actual terms of finishing and polishing. Finishing refers to a comprehensive process and a discrete activity within the overall procedure or process. As a generic concept, finishing and polishing encompass many fields, industries, and applications. In the dental context, the following definitions may be helpful as this article reviews the finishing and polishing of dental restoratives:

- Finishing: the process that involves removing marginal irregularities, defining anatomic contours, and smoothing away surface roughness of a restoration. Finishing includes the process of margination as described below.
- Margination: the specific step of the finishing process that involves the removal of excess restorative material at the junction of the tooth structure and the restorative material, and the application of various finishing techniques to establish a smooth, uniform, and well-adapted cavosurface margin. The resultant junction should conform in shape and normal anatomic characteristics. Optimally, the adjacent natural tooth structure should not be damaged or excessively removed in this procedure. The finish lines of a preparation are often critical to the longevity of many direct and indirect restoratives because forces of polymerization, mastication, and thermal expansion and contraction are transferred to the marginal aspects of the restoration.
- Polishing: the process carried out after the finishing and margination steps of the finishing procedure to remove minute scratches from the surface of a restoration and obtain a smooth, light-reflective luster. The polishing process is also intended to produce a homogeneous surface with minimal microscopic scratches and deflects.

Finishing and polishing in restorative dentistry refers to the steps of (1) gross contouring of the restoration to obtain the desired anatomy, (2) the reduction and smoothing of the surface roughness and scratches created by finishing instruments in the process of gross reduction and initial polishing, and (3) the process of producing a highly smooth, light-reflective, enamel-like surface through final polishing. The dental finishing procedure usually consists of three to four distinct steps or phases involving a number of instruments, as depicted in Fig. 2.

The finishing and polishing procedure involves some fundamental principles that allow us to better understand its application in dentistry. The effectiveness of any finishing or polishing device, and the resultant surface roughness of the restoration, is determined by a number of factors [6,9]:

1. Structure and mechanical properties of the substrate being finished and polished (eg, composite resin, polyacid modified composite resin (so-called "compomer"), glass ionomer, amalgam, porcelain–ceramic materials)
2. Difference in the hardness between the abrasive device and the substrate
3. Particle hardness, size, and shape of abrasive used in the device
4. Physical properties of the backing or bonding material used to carry the abrasive material or substance (eg, rigidity, elasticity, flexibility, thickness, softness, porosity)

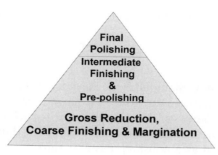

Fig. 2. Finishing and polishing of dental restorative materials encompasses a progression of steps from gross reduction and contouring to final polishing. The "triangle" representation reflects empirical observations regarding the relative amount of time and effort spent on each segment of the process. However, emphasis on aesthetics and surface polish, which has been increasing, may result in greater time and attention to final polishing procedures.

5. Speed and pressure at which the abrasive is applied to the substrate
6. Lubrication and the use of lubricants during the application of the abrasive (eg, water, water-soluble polymers, glycerol, silicon grease, petroleum jelly)

Types and composition of abrasives

Aluminum oxide

Aluminum oxide is a chemical compound of aluminum and oxygen with the chemical formula Al_2O_3. It is also commonly referred to as alumina in the mining, ceramic, and material science disciplines. Its hardness makes it suitable for use as an abrasive and as a component in cutting tools. Aluminum oxide is typically produced as particles bonded to paper or polymer disks and strips or impregnated into rubber wheels and points. It is also the abrasive used for white stones, which consist of sintered aluminum oxide ceramic points of various shapes. Aluminum oxide has sufficient hardness (9 on Mohs' hardness scale) for polishing porcelain, ceramics, and composite resin. Fine particles of aluminum oxide can be mixed into a polishing paste to produce smooth, polished surfaces on many types of restorations, including acrylics and composites.

Carbide compounds

Abrasives in the form of carbide compounds include silicon carbide, boron carbide, and tungsten carbide. The abrading and cutting portion of multifluted finishing burs are manufactured from tungsten carbide bits. Silicon and boron for finishing instruments typically are supplied as particles pressed with a binder into disks, cups, points, or wheels for use on low-piece handpieces. Silicon carbide can also be coated on paper or polymer-backed finishing discs, which are particularly effective for microfilled composite resin restoratives.

Diamond abrasives

Composed of carbon, diamond is the hardest substance known. Diamond is a highly efficient abrasive due to its hardness, thus permitting it to resist wear and maintain sharpness. Diamond dust or particles of various sizes or grits can be coated on a rigid matrix, impregnated within a bonded, elastomeric matrix, or used as a polishing paste or slurry.

Silicon dioxide

Silicon dioxide is used primarily as a polishing agent in bonded abrasive rubber or elastomeric finishing and polishing devices. In dental devices, it is primarily used in rubber or elastomeric cups and points for finishing and polishing. This abrasive is used in the initial finishers and second grit polishers in the Astropol Finishing and Polishing System (Ivoclar North America, Amherst, New York) [4].

Zirconium oxide

Like silicon dioxide, zirconium oxide in dental abrasive devices is used primarily in elastic or rubberlike finishing and polishing rotary shapes. An example of this abrasive is Silicone Points C type (Shofu Dental, Kyoto, Japan), which Watanabe and colleagues [5] report to contain 25 μm zirconium oxide.

Zirconium silicate

Zirconium silicate is a natural mineral often used as a polishing agent in strips, disks, and prophylactic pastes.

Fig. 3 illustrates the broad range of finishing and polishing devices and compositions containing either aluminum oxide or diamond abrasives. These are the two most commonly used abrasives in dentistry and can be surface-bonded on high- or low-rotary burs; impregnated in "rubber," elastomeric bonded abrasive finishers and polishers; or used as loose abrasive polishing pastes.

Table 1 lists the relative hardness of some of these abrasive compounds and lists some examples of their incorporation in various finishing and devices, which the article will now discuss in greater detail.

A review of dental abrasive finishing and polishing devices

A number of methods and tools for finishing and polishing restorations are available to clinicians. These include fluted carbide burs; diamond burs;

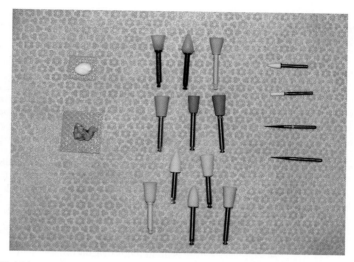

Fig. 3. Finishing and polishing devices and compositions containing aluminum oxide and diamond abrasives. On the upper right-hand side are two rigid bonded abrasive burs, called white stones, which use sintered aluminum oxide. The two devices on the lower right are diamond-coated abrasive burs. On the left are loose abrasive polishing pastes. The white paste on the upper left is aluminum oxide. The gray paste to the lower left is diamond paste. In the center are elastomeric bonded abrasives containing aluminum oxide or diamond particles.

stones; coated abrasive discs and strips; polishing pastes; and soft- or hard-rubber cups, points, and wheels impregnated with various abrasives grits.

Diamond finishing burs

Diamond instruments for dental use were introduced in the United States in 1942, before the introduction and availability of fluted carbide burs [6]. Finishing diamonds are used to contour, adjust, and smooth restorative materials, such as composites and porcelain. Unlike fluted carbide finishing burs (see below), diamond rotary finishing burs rely predominantly on abrasive rather than blade cutting action. These burs have particles of industrial diamonds incorporated into their working surfaces. Diamond instruments consist of three parts: a metal shank or blank, the powdered or particulate diamond abrasive, and a metallic bonding material that bonds the diamond powder onto the shank or blank [6]. They are manufactured in a variety of shapes and sizes and come in different grits, ranging from 7 to 50 μm, depending on the manufacturer. In most cases, they are applied in sequence, starting with a coarser grit and progressing to a finer grit. Diamond burs should always be used with water spray to dissipate heat and at speeds at the lower range of the high-speed turbine. The clinical performance of diamond abrasive instruments depends on such variables as the size, spacing, uniformity, exposure, and bonding of the diamond particles. Diamond

Table 1
Relative hardness values for various dental abrasive compounds, natural tooth structures, and restorative materials [6,9]

Abrasive material	Hardness (Mohs' hardness scale)	Device examples
Diamond	10	Diamond cutting and finishing burs, bonded elastomeric (rubberized) polishers, loose abrasive polishing paste
Silicon carbide	9–10	Coated abrasive finishing–polishing discs
Tungsten carbide	9	Carbide finishing burs
Aluminum oxide	9	White stones, bonded elastomeric (rubberized) finishers–polishers, coated abrasive finishing–polishing discs, loose abrasive polishing paste
Zirconium silicate	7–7.5	Dental prophylaxis paste abrasive
Pumice	6	Dental prophylaxis paste abrasive
Enamel	5	Natural tooth structure
Dentin	3–4	Natural tooth structure
Porcelain	6–7	Restorative material
Gold and gold alloys	2.5–4	Restorative material
Resin composite	5–7	Restorative material
Amalgam	4–5	Restorative material

finishing burs are highly efficient in rates of materials removal, but leave a significantly rough surface, which requires further finishing and polishing [7]. As a result, other finishing and polishing instruments, such as fluted carbide finishing burs, coated abrasive discs, bonded abrasive rubber polishing instruments, and loose abrasive polishing pastes, usually follow the use of diamonds finishing burs. Nevertheless, compared with either aluminum oxide discs or carbide finishing burs, ultrafine finishing diamond burs (40 μm) removed less dentin around the gingival margins of Class V preparations restored with a flowable composite [8].

Carbide finishing burs

Carbide burs are available in a variety of shapes for contouring and finishing. The most commonly used burs have from 8 to 40 fluted blades, and can be straight or twisted. The most common fluted carbide finishing burs have 12, 20, or 40 blades for contouring and smoothing various restorative materials and tooth structures [9]. Carbide finishing burs, due to their less abrasive action, may be kinder to soft tissue at the gingival margin as compared with diamond bur or bonded abrasive contouring instruments. Indirect restorations, such as those using porcelain and other ceramic materials, require specific materials and techniques in finishing and polishing. In an in-vivo evaluation of margin and surface quality with composite and ceramic inlay restorations, initial finishing with a 30-μm diamond followed by finishing with a tungsten carbide finishing bur resulted in a significantly greater amount of continuous margins compared with finishing with two finishing diamonds (20-μm following the 30-μm diamond) [10]. This study suggests the sequential use of carbide finishing burs after use of finishing diamonds for initial contouring and gross reduction to improve surface and marginal quality.

Stones

Dental stones are composed of abrasive particles that have been sintered together or bonded with an organic resin to form a cohesive mass [9]. The color of the stones is an indication of the particular abrasive used: stones containing silicon carbide are green, whereas white stones contain aluminum oxide. The stone is concentrically fixed to the end of a rotary metal shank or blank. Stones are used for contouring and finishing restorations, and have a lower cutting or abrading efficiency than that of diamond burs. Depending on the size of the abrasive grit used, abrasive stones can be provided in coarse, medium, and fine grades of abrasivity.

Coated abrasive finishing and polishing discs and strips

Coated abrasive discs and strips are made by bonding abrasive particles onto a thin polymer or plastic backing [9]. Finishing and polishing discs are used for gross reduction, contouring, finishing, and polishing restorations. The thin layer of abrasive present on these discs remains effective for a limited period of clinical use, making these discs single-use and disposable. Most are coated with an aluminum oxide abrasive, but silicon carbide, garnet, emery, and quartz (cuttle) abrasives are used as well. They are used in a sequence of grits, starting with a coarser grit disc and finishing with a superfine grit. Coated abrasive discs and strips are especially useful on flat or convex surfaces. They work especially well on anterior restorations, such as those involving incisal edges and embrasures, and to a limited extent on posterior composites, especially on interproximal and some buccal–lingual areas. Coated finishing and polishing discs have limited utility on posterior occlusal and concave anterior lingual areas. These areas are better addressed with bond abrasive points and cups, including the newer abrasive-impregnated brushes, which are discussed later in this review.

A number of studies have documented the effectiveness of coated abrasive disc systems [5,11–18]. The range of particle size distributions noted for coated abrasive discs vary from 100 to 55 μm for coarse-grade finishing discs, to 7 to 8 μm for the ultra- or superfine grade of finishing disc [19]. As noted in the studies cited above, coated abrasive discs can finish and provide prepolishing and polishing action for a wide range of restorative materials. Some studies indicate that coated abrasive discs are particularly effective for finishing traditional microfil composite resin materials [11].

Coated abrasive discs are available from a number of manufacturers. These products include the EP Esthetic Polishing System (Brassler), FlexiDisc (Cosmedent), Moore-Flex Polishing System and Moore-Silicon Carbide Discs (E.C. Moore), OptiDisc (Kerr Corporation), Sof-Lex system (3M ESPE), and Super-Snap (Shofu).

Rubber wheels, cups, and points

Rubber polishing instruments are used to finish, smooth, or polish composites. These finishing and polishing instruments are abrasive instruments based on fine or ultrafine hard, abrasive particles dispersed and held in a softer, elastic matrix. The various configurations of these flexible or rubber finishers and polishers complements the access limitations of the coated abrasive discs for such areas as anterior lingual and posterior occlusal surfaces. Shapes, with varying sizes and dimensions, include discs, wheels, cups, and points. Fig. 4 depicts the wide range of bonded, elastomeric finishers–polishers available. They are often sold as kits with a variety of shapes and grits to accommodate the various tooth dimensions and contours presented to the clinician. Flexible, bonded abrasive devices are made by molding abrasive particles of varying particle sizes and size distributions in an elastomeric matrix. The elastomeric matrix can be a natural or synthetic rubber, silicone, or other synthetic elastic polymers. On its labels for Enhance Composite Finishing & Polishing System and Pogo One Step Diamond Micro-Polisher, manufacturer Dentsply/Caulk (Milford, Delaware) lists a patent (U.S. Patent 5,078,754) that describes the use of a "urethane" elastic polymer in which a wide range of abrasive particles can be dispersed, including aluminum oxide and diamond particles [20].

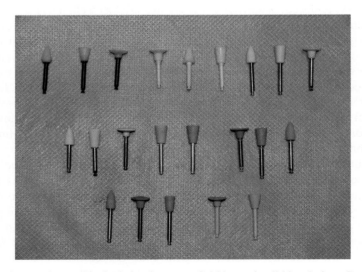

Fig. 4. Elastomeric or rubberized abrasive rotary finishing and polishing devices. Coarser finishing and prepolishing devices are on the top row. Polishing devices are on the lower two rows.

Molded or bonded elastomeric abrasives come in a variety of grits, sizes, shapes, and degrees of firmness. These elastomeric, bonded abrasives are usually molded to a "latch-type" mandrel for slow handpieces. The mandrels are made of stainless steel and high-strength plastic. Some of these products are fabricated to be reusable after sterilization. The abrasives used within these instruments are usually comprised of silicon carbide, aluminum oxide, diamonds, silicon dioxide [4], and zirconium oxide [5]. The particle size distributions listed in the literature range from about 40 μm for an elastomeric aluminum oxide finishing device [5,15,18,21] to 6 μm for a silicone diamond polishing instrument [5,18]. Some of these instruments may be useful in intermediate finishing and in anatomic contouring, as well as prepolishing. Some recent studies have evaluated the efficacy of a variety of bonded, elastomeric abrasive finishers and polishers [4,5, 15,18–24]. Some of the commercial finishing–prepolishing devices (including complete finishing–polishing systems) that appear to have been evaluated in the literature include:

Astropol (Ivoclar Vivadent, Schaan, Liechtenstein) [4,19]
Comprepol and Composhine (Diatech Dental, Heerbrugg, Switzerland) [25]
Enhance (Dentsply/Caulk, Milford, Delaware,) [1,5,12–15,18,19,21]
Flexicups (Cosmedent, Chicago, Illinois) [17]
Identoflex Points (Identoflex AG Buchs, Switzerland) [15]
Identoflex (Kerr Corporation, Orange, California) [24]
Silicone Points C type (Shofu, Kyoto, Japan) [5,18]

Other diamond-containing elastomeric or rubberlike rotary devices have more recently been introduced for finer prepolishing or final polishing. While there appears to be a range of effectiveness in the ability to produce smooth surfaces on direct restorative materials, diamond-impregnated polishers appear particularly effective, with many one- and two-step polishing device systems reaching surface smoothness comparable to multistep, coated-abrasive disc systems. Such diamond one-step polishers that have appeared in some reports include Compomaster (Shofu, Kyoto, Japan) [5,18] and Pogo (Dentsply/Caulk, Milford, Delaware) [21–24]. Diamond-containing polishing devices produce more frictional heat than other bonded-abrasive devices. Hence, to avoid a significant surface-temperature rise that can potentially be deleterious to the restoration as well as to the tooth itself, it is important not to apply heavy pressure when using diamond abrasive rubber polishing instruments.

Loose abrasive polishing pastes and rotary applicator devices for loose abrasives

Loose abrasive polishing pastes are used extensively in industrial and scientific applications [2]. In the three-body, loose abrasive polishing process, the loose abrasive wear induces cutting and ploughing at a micro- and nano-meter scale. Following the example from other industrial and scientific disciplines, dentists have used loose abrasive finishing and polishing compositions for several decades. Loose abrasive polishing pastes used in dental applications are predominantly either based on dispersed and suspended ultrafine aluminum oxide or diamond particles [1]. Aluminum oxide polishing pastes are usually glycerin based with a mean particle size distribution of 1 μm or less. Diamond polishing pastes also use a glycerin-based paste but with a larger mean particle distribution, on the order of 10 μm to <1 μm. Of two diamond polishing pastes mentioned in the literature, one contains diamond particles on the order of 4 to 6 μm and the other contains diamond particles of <1 μm [26]. In this study, which examined the surface morphology and smoothness of the transition from a glass-ceramic insert to a bonded composite resin interface, samples finished with a sequence of progressively smoother diamond abrasive finishing burs (45, 25, and 10 μm), followed by polishing with first a 4- to 6-μm grit diamond polishing paste and then a sub-micrometer diamond polishing paste, exhibited the smoothest transition from composite resin to insert. Of perhaps equal importance, studies and research findings [1,2,27] have indicated that the mode of application and the applicator device's structure and composition can be as important as the composition of the paste used in the polishing procedure. Although the commonly used method for applying polishing paste is the flexible rubber prophy cup, surface roughness data strongly suggest that such a mode of application results in increased surface roughness or, at best, no improvement in surface smoothness. On the other hand, use of soft foam or felt applicators can significantly improve the efficacy of loose abrasive polishing paste, especially those pastes using aluminum oxide as an abrasive. Surface roughness decreased 50% when a 1-μm aluminum oxide polishing paste was applied with a porous synthetic foam cup ($R_a \sim 0.10$), as compared with application of the same paste with a conventional rubber prophy cup ($R_a \sim 0.20$) [27] (R_a refers to "average surface roughness," which is defined as "the arithmetic mean of the absolute values of the profile departures within the sample or evaluation length being measured.").

Fig. 5 depicts the wide range of shapes and sizes of both felt and foam polishing paste applicators, which are optimal for loose abrasive polishing of dental restorations. These applicators can be used with both aluminum-oxide–based and diamond-based polishing pastes.

The technique or mode of applying the polishing paste is also critical. Based on polishing applications in scientific and industrial fields, it is recommended to frequently renew the pad (with fresh polishing paste) and to keep it always wet to prevent crystallization of the colloidal contaminants (such as silica), which can produce scratches [2]. Polishing pastes can probably act in a more aggressive, prepolishing–finishing mode when applied in a dry, anhydrous condition, but also in a polishing mode with the addition of water, facilitating finer abrasive action at nanometer levels on the treated

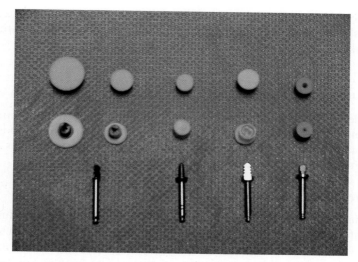

Fig. 5. Synthetic and natural foam or felted polishing paste rotary applicators. These provide a more efficacious and efficient final polishing step using loose abrasive polishing pastes. Synthetic and natural felt applicators are on the left and center. A synthetic foam "cup" applicator is on the far right.

surface. In this mode, polishing pastes tend to produce greater specular reflectance [9], which in turn produces a higher visual surface gloss [12].

With respect to comparative efficacy of polishing pastes as a method for final polishing of composite resins, several investigations report favorable results in producing highly smooth, light-reflective surfaces [5,15,18,28]. These reports involve use of both conventional diamond-stylus contact profilometry, as well as noncontact, three-dimensional surface profile analysis [15]. A differential benefit of polishing paste on various restorative materials has also been noted [19,21], with optimal benefit on a submicrometer, highly filled hybrid material; and surface smoothness equivalent to that obtained through the use of several commercially available bonded abrasive diamond polishing instruments (without the use of polishing paste). Investigations have also noted the benefit of using a loose abrasive, aluminum oxide polishing paste after using sequential, aluminum-oxide–coated abrasive discs for finishing and prepolishing [1,11,27,28]. One investigation has even demonstrated that sequentially applied aluminum oxide polishing pastes produce a visually smooth and light-reflective surface on microfil and small-particle hybrid composites, directly after sequential use of 12-flute and 30- to 40-flute carbide finishing burs [29]. This author has also noted that with careful technique, a finishing–polishing sequence from multifluted carbide burs to sequential polishing pastes is feasible. Nevertheless, others have noted and recommended the need to introduce intermediate finishing and prepolishing devices (eg, coated discs and rubberlike, bonded abrasives) between high-speed contouring–finishing burs and diamonds before the application of polishing pastes for both composite [14] and porcelain [30] restorative materials.

Recent new technology in the realm of dental finishing and polishing

While most new products in the dental finishing and polishing area are "incremental" to existing products, new designs or abrasive compositions periodically appear that raise greater interest and examination. This article highlights two of these recent product technologies.

Abrasive-impregnated brushes and felt devices

Abrasive-impregnated, latch-type polishing brushes were introduced to the professional in the late 1990s. These polishing brushes come in several shapes (pointed, cup-shaped), with a variety of polymer "bristles" impregnated with various abrasive polishing particles. The brushes are intended for reaching into the grooves, fissures, and interproximal areas of ceramic and resin composite restorations that cannot be reached with other finishing or polishing devices without unintended removal of anatomic grooves, fissures, and contours. Several of these brushes are depicted in Fig. 6. The intellectual property literature reveals two US patents that appear specific to this technology [31,32]. Aschmann and Von Weissenfluh [31] describe a "brush

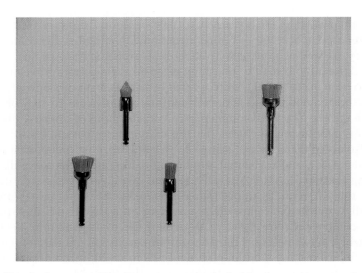

Fig. 6. Abrasive-impregnated brushes, a recent technological development in restorative polishing. The three abrasive brushes from left to right contain diamond particles as the abrasive. The brush on the far right contains silicon carbide.

for surface treatments in restorative dentistry (which) comprises one or several lamellar abrasive elements." Dubbe and Lund [32] describe "a brush for a dental handpiece ... wherein at least some of the bristles comprise an elastomeric material and a number of abrasive particles distributed throughout the elastomeric material." According to 3M ESPE, the company that holds the patent for this brush, the 3M Sof-Lex Brush, the particulate abrasive used in the brush is aluminum oxide [33].

One precursor to this specific abrasive-impregnated brush technology appears to have been diamond-impregnated felt wheels for polishing a hybrid composite resin [34]. These diamond-impregnated felt wheels appeared effective in smoothing the surface of a hybrid composite resin after initial finishing with various sequences of high-speed diamond burs, tungsten carbide finishing burs, or combinations of diamond and carbide finishing burs. In 1999, an early report on these new polishing devices [31] described the evaluation of a new polishing brush, Occlubrush (Hawe-Neos, now Kerr Corporation, a division of Danaher Corporation, Orange, California), composed of rigid polycarbonate fibers impregnated with silicon carbide abrasive particles. The investigators found that the silicon-carbide–impregnated bristle polishing brush maintained surface texture during the polishing procedure, produced a composite surface smoothness somewhere between that created by a 25-μm finishing diamond and a extra-fine coated abrasive disc, provided a surface luster subjectively greater than an extra-fine coated abrasive disc (on composite resin and enamel), could be reused with autoclaving 15 to 19 times, and was no more deleterious to enamel surface quality or restoration marginal quality than a 25-μm finishing diamond.

More recently, a few in-vitro evaluations have assessed the polishing efficacy of these abrasive-impregnated polishing brushes. Yap and colleagues [22,23] evaluated the residual surface roughness after use of the Sof-Lex Brush (3M ESPE, St. Paul, Minnesota) and found that the brush produced a smooth, polished surface comparable to that following the use of a rubber or bonded abrasive diamond polishing device. Venturini and colleagues [17] evaluated a silicon-carbide–impregnated polishing brush, the Jiffy Polishing Brush (Ultradent, South Jordan, Utah), after finishing–prepolishing with sequential rubber polishing cups (Flexicups/Cosmodent). They found a high level of surface smoothness in both microfilm and hybrid composite resins after polishing with this impregnated brush for both an immediate and a delayed polishing technique. This polishing device design is interesting in its approach to providing improved "micro-access" for bonded abrasive polishing, and needs further laboratory and clinical evaluation.

Rotary resin-matrix stain, cement, composite removing devices

Several rotary devices based on a polymer or composite resin binder or matrix, with apparent "controlled" abrasivity, have recently been introduced to selectively remove surface-adherent restorative materials, including composite resin and residual cement. Examples of this new class of abrasive devices includes StainBuster (Danville, San Ramon, California; and Carbotech, Ganges, France), a latch-type, rotary composite fiber bur that Danville claims will remove residual composite with no damage to either enamel or porcelain. Other stated intended uses, according to the company, include removal of residual orthodontic adhesive, periodontal root planing, and stain removal on tooth structure for areas with limited access. This specific product is apparently manufactured by Carbotech under US Patent 6,386,874 [35], according to the package label. The patent abstract indicates that the structure of the "rod" bur "is made up of fibers and optionally a load of particles embedded in a resinous matrix giving the working surface of the rod a continuous abrasive power." The primary claim (Claim 1) listed in the patent is:

> Hygiene instrument for the cleaning and polishing of the surface of teeth and/or composite materials of dental fillings, said instrument having the shape of a rod, the structure of which comprises fibers embedded in a resinous matrix wherein the fibers are made from a glass enriched with zirconium oxide, giving to the instrument a high resistance to at least one of an alkaline and acidic agent and making the instrument detectable by electromagnetic radiation.

The other new product in this class is OptiClean (Kerr Dental, a division of Danaher Corporation, Orange, California), a latch-type rotary

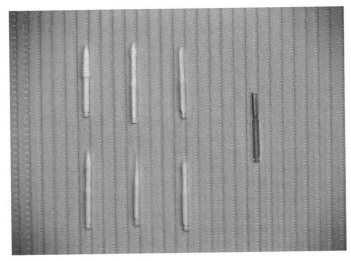

Fig. 7. Recent rotary finishing–polishing devices. The white, fiber-impregnated polymer rotary burs have been suggested and indicated for "minimally" abrasive action (ie, stain removal, selective composite removal). The blue rotary bur (*right*) is suggested for removal and cleaning of temporary cement on tooth preparations before final cementation.

bur composed of aromatic polyamide containing 40-μm aluminum oxide. According to the manufacturer, OptiClean is intended for removal of temporary cement and debris on tooth preparations before final cementation and therefore replaces other methods of preparation surface cleaning, such as a rubber cup and pumice, or use of hand instruments. The manufacture lists US Patent 5,882,201 on its labeling for the product [36]. This patent details a rotary dental bur, of a specific dimension and composition, intended to be used to "remove a surface contaminant from a surface of a tooth." Both of these products, which are depicted in Fig. 7, await further independent studies and evaluations to more fully understand their performance.

Summary

The primary goal of finishing and polishing technology and procedures in dental restorative procedures is to create restorations that are aesthetically natural and harmonize both in function and appearance with the surrounding natural tooth structure. Highly effective and efficient finishing and polishing procedures achieve this objective by producing restorations with a surface smoothness and light reflectivity similar to natural tooth structure. Optimal surface properties and smoothness are also important for maintaining the tooth-restorative interface-appropriate oral hygiene procedures. This article provides a clinically useful, outcome-supported discussion of existing and well-known products, and also provides a glimpse into new and emerging concepts in optimal surface finishing, polishing, and surface maintenance in restorative dentistry.

References

[1] Jefferies SR. The art and science of abrasive finishing and polishing in restorative dentistry. Dent Clin North Am 1998;42:613–27.

[2] Remond G, Nockolds C, Philips M, et al. Implications of polishing techniques in quantitative x-ray microanalysis. J Res Natl Inst Stand Technol 2002;107:639–62.

[3] Jones CS, Billington RW, Peason GJ. Interoperator variability during polishing. Quintessence Int 2006;37(3):183–90.

[4] U.S. Air Force Dental Evaluation & Consultation Service, 61–19 Astropol Finishing and Polishing System (Project 00-13). Available at: https://decs.nhgl.med.navy.mil/Dis61/sec12.htm.

[5] Watanabe T, Miyazaki M, Takamizawa T, et al. Influence of polishing duration on surface roughness of resin composites. J Oral Sci 2005;47:21–5.

[6] Bayne SC, Thompson JY, Sturdevant CM, et al. Sturdevant's art & science of operative dentistry. In: Roberson TM, Heymann HO, Swift EJ, editors. Chaper 7: instruments and equipment for tooth preparation. St. Louis: Mosby; 2002. p. 307–44.

[7] Jung M. Surface roughness and cutting efficiency of composite finishing instruments. Oper Dent 1997;22(2):98–104.

[8] Mitchell CA, Pintado MR, Douglas WH. Iatrogenic tooth abrasion comparisons among composite materials and finishing techniques. J Prosthet Dent 2002;88(3):320–8.

[9] O'Brien WJ. Dental materials and their selection. In: O'Brien WJ, editor. Chapter 10: abrasion, polishing, and bleaching. Chicago: Quintessence Books; 2002. p. 156–64.

[10] Jung M, Wehlen O, Klimek J. Finishing and polishing of indirect composite and ceramic inlays in-vivo: occlusal surfaces. Oper Dent 2004;29(2):131–41.

[11] Jefferies SR, Smith RL, Barkmeier WW, et al. Comparison of surface smoothness of restorative resin materials. J Esthet Dent 1989;1:169–75.

[12] Hondrum SO, Fernández R Jr. Contouring, finishing, and polishing Class V restorative materials. Oper Dent 1997;22(1):30–6.

[13] Yap AUJ, Lye KW, Sau CW. Surface characteristics of tooth-colored restoratives polished utilizing different polishing systems. Oper Dent 1997;22(3):260–5.

[14] Hoelscher DC, Neme AM, Pink FE, et al. The effect of three finishing systems on four esthetic restorative materials. Oper Dent 1998;23(1):36–42.

[15] Marigo L, Rizzi M, LaTorre G, et al. 3-D surface profile analysis: different finishing methods for resin composites. Oper Dent 2001;26:562–8.

[16] Üçtaşli MB, Bala O, Güllü A. Surface roughness of flowable and packable composite resin materials after finishing with abrasive discs. J Oral Rehabil 2004;31:1197–202.

[17] Venturini D, Cenci MS, Demarco FF, et al. Effect of polishing technique and time on surface roughness, hardness and microleakage of resin composite restorations. Oper Dent 2006; 31(1):11–7.

[18] Watanabe T, Miyazaki M, Moore BK. Influence of polishing instruments on the surface texture of resin composites. Quintessence Int 2006;37(1):61–7.

[19] Gedik R, Hürmüzlü F, Coşkun A, et al. Surface roughness of new microhybrid resin-based composites. J Am Dent Assoc 2005;136(8):1106–12.

[20] Jefferies SR, Smith RL, Green RD. Finishing/polishing system. US Patent 5,078,754. January 7, 1992.

[21] Türkün LS, Türkün M. The effect of one-step polishing system on the surface roughness of three esthetic resin composite materials. Oper Dent 2004;29(2):203–11.

[22] Yap AUJ, Yap SH, Teo CK, et al. Finishing/polishing of composite and compomer restoratives: effectiveness of one-step systems. Oper Dent 2004;29(4):275–9.

[23] Yap AUJ, Ng JJ, Yap SH, et al. Surface finish of resin-modified and highly viscous glass ionomer cements produced by new one-step systems. Oper Dent 2004;29(1):87–91.

[24] St-Georges AJ, Bolla M, Fortin D, et al. Surface finish produced on three resin composites by new polishing systems. Oper Dent 2005;30(5):593–7.

[25] Özgünaltay G, Yazici AR, Görücü J. Effect of finishing and polishing procedures on the surface roughness of new tooth-coloured restoratives. J Oral Rehabil 2003;30: 218–24.

[26] Ashe MJ, Tripp GA, Eichmiller FC, et al. Surface roughness of glass-ceramic insert-composite restorations: assessing several polishing techniques. J Am Dent Assoc 1996;127(10): 1495–500.

[27] Jefferies SR, Smith RL, Barkmeier WW, et al. Benefit of polishing pastes on various resin composites [abstract 1006]. J Dent Res 1991;70(spec iss):291.

[28] Turssi CP, Saad JRC, Duarte SLL, et al. Composite surfaces after finishing and polishing techniques. Am J Dent; 13(3):136–8.

[29] Boghosian AA, Randolph RG, Jekkals VJ. Rotary instrument finishing of microfilled and small-particle hybrid composite resins. J Am Dent Assoc 1987;115:299–301.

[30] Al-Wahadni A. An in-vitro investigation into the surface roughness of 2 glazed, unglazed, and refinished ceramic materials. Quintessence Int 2006;37(4):311–7.

[31] Aschmann F, Von Weissenfluh BA. Brush for use in restorative dentistry. US Patent 6,312,257. November 6, 2001.

[32] Dubbe JW, Lund YI. Dental handpiece brush and method of using the same. US Patent 6,554,614. April 29, 2003.

[33] 3M ESPE. 3M Worldwide. Available at: http://www.3m.com/espe. Accessed December 16, 2006.

[34] Krejci I, Lutz F, Boretti R. Resin composite polishing—filling the gaps. Quintessence Int 1999;30(7):490–5.
[35] Bachmann MW, Bachmann S, Bachmann N. Hygiene instrument for cleaning and polishing the surface of the teeth and the composite materials of dental filings, in the shape of a rod. US Patent 6,386,874. May 14, 2002.
[36] Salem G. Dental debridement method and tool therefore. US Patent 5,882,201. March 16, 1999.

ELSEVIER
SAUNDERS

Dent Clin N Am 51 (2007) 399–417

THE DENTAL
CLINICS
OF NORTH AMERICA

Porcelain Laminate Veneers: Reasons for 25 Years of Success

John R. Calamia, DMD[a],*,
Christine S. Calamia, DDS[b]

[a]*Department of Cariology and Comprehensive Care, New York University College of Dentistry, 345 East 24th Street, New York, NY 10010-4086, USA*
[b]*Department of Biomaterials and Biomemetics, New York University College of Dentistry, New York, NY*

Since its introduction more than two decades ago [1,2], etched porcelain veneer restoration has proved to be a durable and aesthetic modality of treatment [3–6]. These past 25 years of success can be attributed to great attention to detail in the following areas: (1) planning the case, (2) conservative (enamel saving) preparation of teeth, (3) proper selection of ceramics to use, (4) proper selection of the materials and methods of cementation of these restorations, (5) proper finishing and polishing of the restorations, and (6) proper planning for the continuing maintenance of these restorations. This article discusses failures that could occur if meticulous attention is not given to such details. Failures that did occur structurally and aesthetically warned individuals who were learning the procedure what to watch for. Some concerns as to newer products and methods and their effect on the continued success of this modality of treatment are also addressed.

Shade matching

Aesthetic shade matching and masking with thin porcelain veneer restorations are arguably the most demanding facets of this procedure. The key to success is understanding that the final color obtained is a combined metamerism of the tooth, the resin cement selected, and the porcelain used for the restoration.

---

* Corresponding author.
E-mail address: jrc1@nyu.edu (J.R. Calamia).

0011-8532/07/$ - see front matter © 2007 Published by Elsevier Inc.
doi:10.1016/j.cden.2007.03.008   *dental.theclinics.com*

The first part of the equation—the underlying tooth—can play a crucial role in the final appearance of the restoration. Imperfections should be minimized, and existing restorations should be changed either before preparation and impression making or at the time of insertion. The clinician also may try to change the color of the teeth to be veneered (ie, tetracycline-stained case) with the use of modern bleaching techniques [7]. The final opacity, translucency, and distribution of color of the existing tooth (the stump shade) should be communicated thoroughly to the technician by intraoral photographs, shade drawings, and custom shade guides to allow the technician to plan the most important part of the equation, the final restoration. Masking undesirable discolorations without sacrificing natural translucency in the final restoration requires technical skills and experienced workmanship that can only be tapped if the technician receives enough information about the case. Using contemporary feldspathic porcelain (Omega900, Vident, Brea, CA; Finesse, Dentsply Prosthetic, York, PA; IPS, D.Sign, Ivoclar Vivadent, Amherst, NY) and metal-free, high-strength restorations (IPS Empress, D.Sign, Ivoclar Vivadent, Amherst, NY; OPC, Pentron Laboratories, Wallingford, CT), which are developed specifically for bonded restorations, dental laboratory professionals are able to vary translucency and internal characterizations in the fabrication of aesthetic restorations. The technician's experience and ability are of vital importance to a successful case.

The last component of the equation is the luting cement. Under normal circumstances, the cement is probably the least responsible for the final result obtained, contributing less than 10% of the final color of the restoration. There is an important contribution, however. Generally, the higher the filler content of cement, the more refractive and opaque the final color of the restoration. If the laboratory technician incorporates a spacer on the die on which the veneer is fabricated, this important component of the process can be addressed. The resultant increase in distance between the tooth and the veneer allows for increased control of the restoration color with resin cement. The value and opacity of the underlying cement are generally more important than the hue or chroma selected [8]. It is the authors' experience that thin viscosity, highly filled resin cements cause fewer long-term problems with marginal discoloration and air entrapment than do more viscous resin formulations. Recent-generation resin cements (eg, Calibra, Dentsply Caulk, Milford, DE; Choice II, Bisco, Schaumburg, IL; Lutelt, Pentron Corp., Wallingford, CT; Variolink I and Appeal, Ivoclar Vivadent, Amherst, NY; Ultra Bond Improved, Den-Mat Corp., Santa Monica, CA) can be light cured or, if used with thick restorations such as inlays, onlays, or crowns, dual cured with the addition of catalyst added to the base cement. It should be noted that once the dual-cure component is added, the likelihood exists that the restoration may change slightly in color over time because of the aromatic tertiary amine component of dual-cure products [9–11]. Dual cure resin cement use should be limited to posterior restorations outside the smile line.

In instances in which classes III and IV restorations that require replacement are in contact with the veneer preparation, the authors also had success with microhybrid restorative resins used as cements (ie, TPH Spectrum, Dentsply Caulk, Milford, DE; Venus, Heraeus Kulzer, Armonk, NY; Point 4 Sybron/Kerr, Orange, CA). These resin cements are opaque enough that they are also useful in masking stained teeth (ie, tetracycline-stained cases). Clinicians should take care to properly provide a better contact angle of these more highly viscose materials to the veneer. This is accomplished by first applying a thin layer of a light-cured unfilled resin to the veneer and then syringing the hybrid directly on the intaglio (ie, internal surface) of the restoration. A composite instrument is used to flatten the hybrid over the surface so that no air is trapped. The restoration should be seated slowly and with pressure to ensure complete seating. Any excess resin cement is removed with a microbrush soaked with unfilled resin. Finally, the veneer is pushed into place one last time. Excess resin is left in place to ensure that there are no voids at the margins. While slight finger pressure is applied, the restoration is cured for at least 5 seconds with a standard halogen or LED light, after which finger pressure is no longer needed and the curing of the resin cement is continued for additional 40 seconds. These restorations cannot be overcured, so more curing time is better than less curing time.

Marginal discoloration and loss of color stability

The least common problems associated with porcelain laminate veneers are marginal discoloration and loss of color stability. These problems seldom occur because (1) all margins are in cleansable areas often easily finished and polished at the time of cementation and (2) the glazed porcelain surface, which is mostly impervious to extrinsic stain, also protects underlying light-cured (more color stable) resin cement [10].

If a well-fitted restoration has been returned and a thin viscosity, but highly filled, resin cement has been used with proper finishing and polishing techniques, immediate marginal discoloration is rare, and little or no marginal discoloration is usually seen at long-term follow-up. However, ill-fitting veneers, which expose inappropriate amounts of resin cement at their margins, or well-fitting but poorly seated restorations caused by the use of highly viscous cements often show a dark line stain at the margins (Fig. 1). Only refinishing and repolishing can remove these dark lines. If these lines are too deep, then a replacement restoration may be necessary. To remove excess cement, the author uses a series of trimming diamonds (ie, ET, Brasseler USA, Savannah, GA) in a 30-μm, 15-μm, and 8-μm sequence of finishing diamonds. (The Two-Striper MFS, another kit of diamond finishing instruments by Premier Dental, Plymouth Meeting, PA, comes in 40-μm, 20-μm, and 10-μm series.) This process is followed by

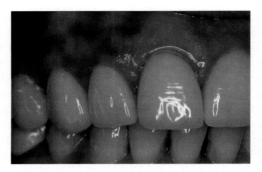

Fig. 1. Clinical view of discolored line that results from improper finishing or an undercontoured margin.

finishing and polishing with strips and disks (ie, Sof-Lex, 3M Espe, St. Paul, MN) and then by porcelain diamond polishing paste applied with rubber cups.

Breakdown in bonds

A possible cause of marginal discoloration and the loss of color stability of the restoration is marginal leakage or a breakdown of the bond either between the cement and the tooth or between the cement and the veneer. This discoloration starts as a dark line but eventually works its way under the restoration, with a resultant diffused discoloration that spreads from the involved margin. This phenomenon was common with acrylic laminate veneers as a result of the poor bond strength at the cement and acrylic veneer interface. This separation is uncommon for porcelain veneers because under normal circumstances, the bond to porcelain by the cement and the bond of composite cement to tooth is more than acceptable to retain the veneer over the long-term [12,13].

However, if the veneer is not properly etched or if the veneer and tooth are in some way contaminated during the bonding process (ie, water or oil in the air lines), it is possible to experience this problem or worse—the complete delamination of the veneer. This occurrence is rare, and it is usually important to pay close attention to the porcelain, composite, and tooth interfaces (Figs. 2 and 3). Organization of steps at the time of bonding usually eliminates this concern. If a debonded but good-fitting restoration is recovered, the tooth may be cleaned of all old composite using magnification. The intaglio of the restoration intern can be delicately sandblasted and re-etched using hydrofluoric acid and then cleaned, silanated, and recemented.

Air bubble entrapment

Air bubbles can become entrapped near the margin of the restoration, which eventually becomes exposed. Food and other debris may be packed

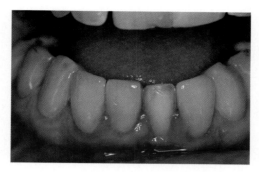

Fig. 2. Delamination of tooth #24 is caused by poor cementation. Excess resin cement is also present at the cervical margin of tooth #27 and is subgingival on teeth #23 through #25, causing excessive gingival irritation.

into the small space between the restoration and the tooth. Although this is a rare occurrence, the best treatment is first gaining proper access to this void with a pointed diamond and thoroughly removing any food and debris impaction. The porcelain can be etched with mild hydrofluoric acid and silanated, the tooth can be etched with 37% phosphoric acid, and a new resin cement can be introduced with a thin syringe tip or compule.

Leaking, old restorations or an uncovered surface of the veneered tooth also may cause generalized discoloration. This possibility should be examined, and if it is found to be the cause of any discoloration, the restoration should be removed and restored (Figs. 4 and 5). There has been some speculation that dual-cured or chemically cured composite resins used as cements for veneers eventually can discolor over time, with resultant change of veneer color. Modern porcelain veneer cements are generally packaged as base shades only and are light cured. Some of these cements can be used in conjunction with the appropriate catalyst to be used as dual cements,

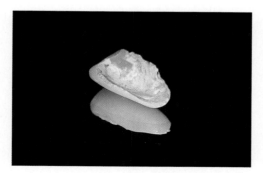

Fig. 3. It is evident from this debonded restoration that contamination occurred at the interface between the cement and the tooth surface. Almost all of the cement is still attached to the veneer.

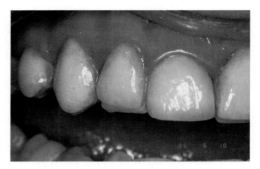

Fig. 4. Improperly placed laminates are positioned too cervically, which is primarily caused by little or no preparation of the teeth and no positive lock into place.

but they should have limited use on posterior restorations outside the smile line.

Cohesive failure and repair

Another rare occurrence is the cohesive failure of either the tooth or the porcelain. In the first instance, the fracture of the underlying tooth is usually the result of poor judgment in selection of the tooth to be veneered. Vital anterior teeth with large existing restorations on the mesial and distal surfaces might be better served with full-coverage porcelain restorations bonded to the additional surface area of the crown preparation on dentin. Nonvital anterior teeth that have at least one surface with large existing restoration and an average-to-large lingual access from root canal therapy should be considered for post core and full-coverage porcelain crowns (Figs. 6 and 7) [2,3].

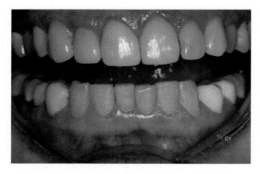

Fig. 5. Leakage of a restoration on the mesiolingual surface of tooth #10 resulted in a discoloration of its mesiofacial surface. Excess cement is also visible at the mesiocervical of tooth #6. Poor axial inclination is also evident on teeth #9, 10, 11.

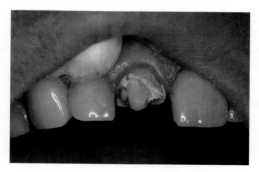

Fig. 6. Buccal view of fractured tooth with large access opening for root canal therapy and a large mesiolingual class III restoration. Placement of an esthetic post and full coverage might have been a better choice.

A more common problem is the cohesive failure of the porcelain itself, which may occur during cementation as a result of a poor-fitting restoration, a resin that is too thick (viscous), or a resin that has gone through some initial setting. The latter can result if the resin is left too long in ambient light or unit light. Cohesive failure also may occur after cementation as the result of poorly planned occlusion or traumatic injury. It is important to note that these fractures, after cementation, occur almost exclusively within porcelain and rarely extend to the junction of porcelain and cement. In the case of veneer fractured at the time of placement, the restoration still may be placed temporarily because of the usual intimate fit of the pieces. The patient is informed of the problem and an appointment is made for removal of the fractured veneer and creation of an impression for its final replacement. This scenario has occurred twice in the authors' experience, and in both instances the patients did not see any aesthetic difference in the fractured restoration compared with other restorations. To date, both patients have not elected to have the fractured restorations replaced. One such case is 12 years old and

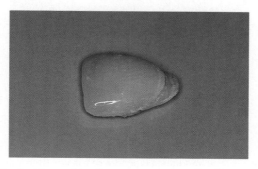

Fig. 7. It is interesting that the resulting fracture occurred totally within the tooth and the bond between the veneer and the facial enamel remains intact.

the other is 8 years old. Since we began using high-strength porcelains, no further fractures on placement have been experienced.

In the case of restorations that experience cohesive failure after cementation, repair may be attempted depending on the extent of the fracture. The following steps are suggested to follow for this type of repair.

1. A rubber dam should be applied. Resin block-out materials, similar to those used to protect gingival tissue during bleaching procedures, also can be used if a small area is involved but control of the field is necessary. At least cotton roll isolation and high-speed evacuation are warranted.
2. Sandblasting of the area to be etched is suggested, generally with 50-μm aluminum oxide particles. Roughening of the porcelain at the margin with a coarse diamond may suffice.
3. Hydrofluoric acid is applied to the roughened porcelain surface (Fig. 8), which is followed by the placement of phosphoric acid on exposed dentin and/or enamel.
4. After following the manufacturer's directions on etch time, one should rinse and dry the surface.
5. A suitable silane coupling agent is applied to the porcelain only (Fig. 9).

Premixed silanes generally have a short shelf life and should be used as soon as possible. Silanes that come in two bottles that require mixing are generally best. Silanes are transferred to the surface of the porcelain in a chemical vehicle that dissipates on drying. Care should be used to ensure that the treated surface is dried properly. If the chemical vehicle is still present (usually indicated by a wet appearance on the surface), it could act as a separating medium and, rather than boost the bond strength, cause delamination. It is important to follow manufacturer instructions exactly [14–16].

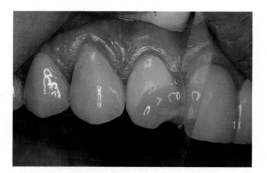

Fig. 8. Repair of the porcelain restoration is performed conservatively using an adhesive bonding protocol. Here the porcelain has been roughened, and hydrofluoric acid was placed to etch porcelain intraorally. Exposed tooth is etched with phosphoric acid.

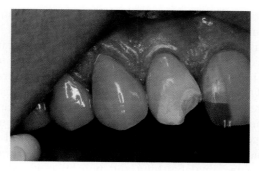

Fig. 9. The acids are removed with a water spray and dried. A silane coupling agent is applied and allowed to dry thoroughly. The properly etched and silanated surface is evident.

After the silane has been added and dried, an appropriate unfilled resin or dentin bonding agent may be added to the porcelain/tooth interface and the excess is blown off the surface to be repaired. This process prevents the pooling of unfilled resin, which weakens the repair. This unfilled resin-covered surface is then light cured for at least 20 seconds. Finally, a filled hybrid or micro-filled composite is placed, appropriately contoured, and cured as the repair material. It may be finished and polished to provide a smooth surface (Fig. 10). In the short-term, it is difficult to delineate where the repair material has been placed, but in the long-term, a new restoration eventually may need to be considered.

Improper occlusion and its periodontal implications

Because most porcelain veneers are fabricated on the facial surface of maxillary anterior teeth, occlusion is often not considered critical to the success of these cases. On the contrary, occlusion is of vital importance, not

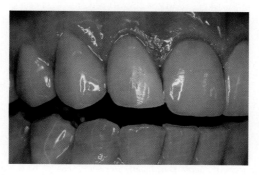

Fig. 10. An unfilled composite resin is applied, air thinned, and cured. This process is followed by application of microhybrid composite resin for an aesthetic—yet durable—repair.

only in vertical occlusion but also in lateral and protrusive movements. Even a slight lengthening of the maxillary anterior teeth over the incisal edge can have severe consequences on the unrestored mandibular dentition because of the difference in hardness between porcelain and the natural enamel. This difference becomes even more critical in canine and first premolar occlusion (Fig. 11). In some isolated cases, the author also has observed unusual gingival recession patterns in teeth that may have been inadvertently brought into increased occlusal stress after lamination. If occlusion is not properly planned into the final restorations, it likely will result in long-term consequences. All cases should be articulated and checked carefully before insertion, and final finishing and polishing should follow occlusal equilibration followed by protective night guard appliances.

Discussion

The etched porcelain veneer has proved to be one of the most successful modalities of treatment that modern dentistry has to offer. Difficulties with this restoration have been relatively nonexistent over the past 25 years. The problems that have arisen seem to involve matters of proper patient selection, attention to details in preparation and final placement, and material and laboratory selection. The latest resin cements, bonding agents, and high-strength ceramics have expanded the etched porcelain technology for inlays, onlays, crowns, and simple bridges (Figs. 12–14).

With the advent of new dentin-bonding agents, ceramics that required more room in preparation to allow for processing (ie, pressed ceramics), and failure of many to take advantage of multidisciplinary cases incorporating orthodontics, oral surgery, and endodontics, however, the key concept of the preservation of enamel somehow has gone by the wayside or been considered less important. This may be a huge mistake. Deeper preparation into dentin, a substrate that has a much lower modulus of

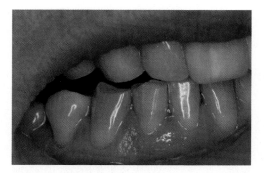

Fig. 11. Porcelain veneers on facial-incisal teeth #6 and #7 seem to be wearing the facial-incisal of teeth #26 and #27. Restoration of the occluding mandibular teeth should have been considered in this case.

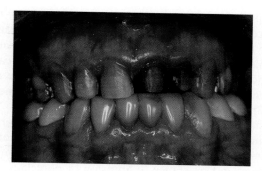

Fig. 12. In this tetracycline case, the existing composite bonding is removed and the teeth are prepared for porcelain veneers and full-coverage porcelain crowns.

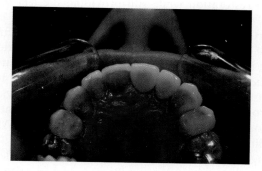

Fig. 13. Incisal/occlusal view of seated maxillary restorations. Note the natural arch form and harmony of the definitive restorations.

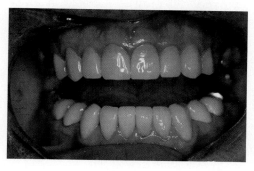

Fig. 14. Postoperative facial view of the definitive all-ceramic veneer and crown restorations.

elasticity than porcelain, has provided a less rigid base or foundation for restoration placement than enamel. This approach has resulted in reports of much higher fracture rates than other previous enamel supported restorations [17]. This disturbing trend has been further complicated by the use of self-etch bonding agents that may show more long-term degradation of the dentinal bond because of water permeations at the adhesive dentin interphase [18–22].

Over the past 25 years, the etched porcelain-bonded restoration has demonstrated four important criteria, in the opinion of the authors, in determining the ultimate success of this dental restorative system: (1) adequate strength, hardness, and resistance to abrasion of porcelain exo-skin, which protects the resin adhesive undercoating, (2) biocompatibility with—but resistance to—the oral environment of the total restoration, (3) ability to be formed into the necessary shapes and colors while retaining the tooth's natural translucency, and (4) values for thermal conductivity and coefficient of thermal expansion, similar to that of tooth structure, allowing long-term adhesion of the restoration while still providing the feel of natural tooth surface.

These important characteristics must place porcelain laminate veneers among the most successful restorations that dentistry provides. This modality of treatment has been part of the curriculum in only a few dental schools in North America, which has given rise to many privately owned institutes being happy to fill this gap in modern education and providing what they consider the proper techniques and philosophy of treatment using this restoration. It is our hope that all dental schools in North America will see value in providing the proper training to their students.

The following case handled at New York University College of Dentistry by a fourth-year student incorporated 20 all-porcelain restorations. The result was a revitalized smile of a young female executive (Figs. 15–18).

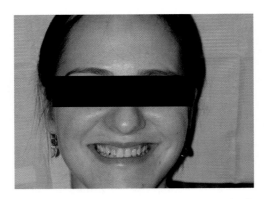

Fig. 15. Unattractive smile with leaking restoration and yellow teeth.

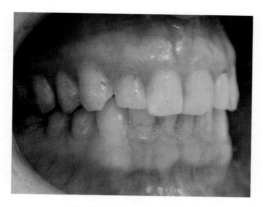

Fig. 16. Right lateral view.

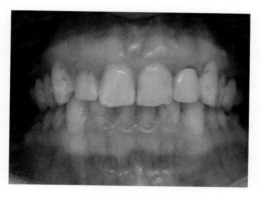

Fig. 17. Direct frontal view.

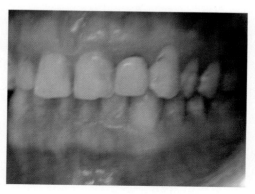

Fig. 18. Left lateral view. Poor crown margin.

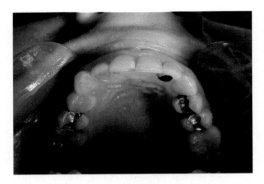

Fig. 19. Maxillary incisal/occlusal view.

Based on radiographs and an intraoral examination, it was clear that the patient is at high risk for caries. All premolars had existing amalgam or composite restorations. All incisors had large mesial and distal restorations. Some of these restorations contained open margins. The patient's main complaint was that she would like all her teeth to be the same shade and not cracked. She did feel that her teeth appeared too small (Figs. 19–21). After exploring all possibilities, a treatment plan was decided on and agreed to by the patient:

1) The premolar restorations would be restored with composite.
2) Tooth #10 had an existing porcelain fused to metal crown that, with time, had caused gingival recession. It would be replaced with an all porcelain crown.
3) Teeth #4–6, 11–13, 20–22, 27–29 would be restored with a feldspathic porcelain (soft spar veneers).
4) Teeth #7–10 and 23–26 would be restored with (soft spare) porcelain crowns to provide full coverage to incisors with large restorations of endodontically treated teeth (Figs. 22–30).

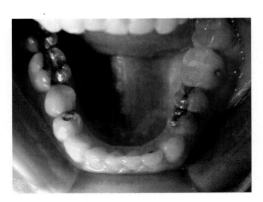

Fig. 20. Mandibular incisal/occlusal view.

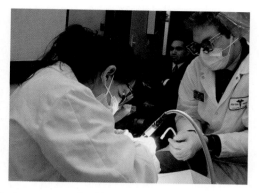

Fig. 21. NYU student prepares teeth while another student assists. In this way, two students can share the knowledge of one large case.

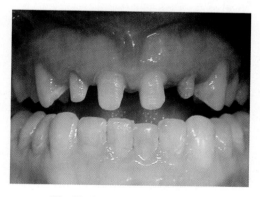

Fig. 22. Prepared maxillary teeth.

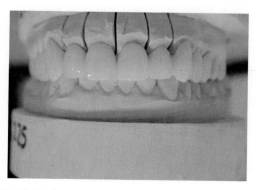

Fig. 23. Finished restorations on working cast, direct facial view.

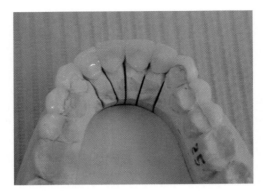

Fig. 24. Finished restorations on working cast, palatal view.

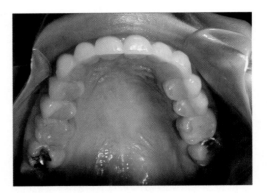

Fig. 25. Finished maxillary restorations, palatal view.

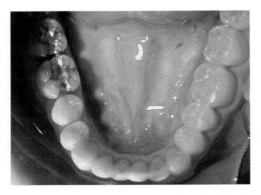

Fig. 26. Finished mandibular restorations, incisal view.

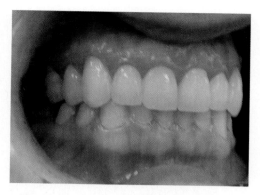

Fig. 27. Finished restorations, left lateral view.

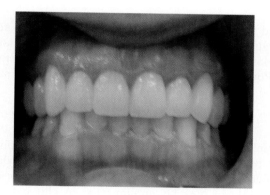

Fig. 28. Finished restorations, direct view.

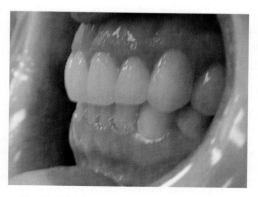

Fig. 29. Finished restorations, left lateral view.

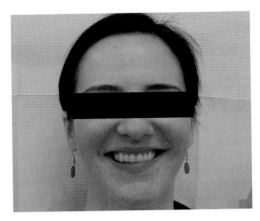

Fig. 30. Improved smile.

All prepared teeth were etched with a 35% phosphoric acid, and prime and bond bonding agent was applied. Softspar crowns and veneers were treated with silane and cemented to teeth with Vario-link transparent base resin cement. Pogo polishing cones were used to polish the final restorations.

Summary

Etched porcelain veneer technology has demonstrated long-term clinical success. It has proved to be one of the most successful modalities of treatment that modern dentistry has to offer. The relatively few difficulties that have been encountered may be circumvented or eliminated if the practitioner pays close attention to detail. Development of new products and materials is expected to bring longer term success. Modern-day restorations offer great promise for the expanded use of the etched porcelain/resin-bonded system for inlays, onlays, crowns, and simple bridges if the ability of bonding to dentin is respected and further researched. Evidence based principals need to determined and followed, like what has been done with porcelain veneer bonding to enamel.

References

[1] Calamia, John R. Etched porcelain facial veneers: a new treatment modality. N Y J Dent Sept 1983;53:255–9.
[2] Horn H. A new lamination, porcelain bonded to enamel. N Y State Dent J 1983;49(6):401–3.
[3] Nathanson D, Strassler HE. Clinical evaluation of etched porcelain veneers over a period of 18 to 42 months. J Esthet Dent 1984;1(1):21–8.
[4] Calamia JR. Clinical evaluation of etched porcelain veneers. Am J Dent Feb 1989;2(1).
[5] Strassler HS, Weiner S. Long-term clinical evaluation of etched porcelain veneers [abstract 1017]. J Dent Res (special issue) 1998;233.

[6] Friedman MJ. A 15 year review of porcelain veneer failure—a clinician's observations. Compend Contin Educ Dent 1998;19:625–36.

[7] Strassler HE, Calamia JR, Scherer W. An update on carbamide peroxide at home bleaching agents. N Y State Dent J April 1992;30–5.

[8] Calamia JR. Etched porcelain veneers: the current state of the art [abstract 1154]. Quintessence Int 1985;16(1):5–12.

[9] Noie F, O'Keefe KL, Powers JM. Color stability of resin cements after accelerated aging. Int J Prosthodont 1995;8(1):51–5.

[10] Hekimoglu C, Anil N, Etikan I. Effect of accelerated aging on the color stability of cemented laminate veneers. Int J Prosthodont 2000;13(1):29–33.

[11] Nathanson D, Bansar F. Color stability of resin cements- an in vivo study. Pract Proced Aesthet Dent 2002;14(6):449–55.

[12] Simonsen RJ, Calamia JR. Tensile bond strengths of etched porcelain [abstract 1154]. J Dent Res 1983;62:297.

[13] Calamia JR, Simonsen RJ. Effect of coupling agents on bond strength of etched porcelain [abstract 79]. J Dent Res March 1984;63:179.

[14] Plueddemann EP. Adhesion through silane coupling agents. Fundamentals of Adhesion. New York: Plenum press; 1991. p. 279–90.

[15] Soderholm KJ, Shanq SW. Molecular orientation of silane at the surface of colloidal silica. J Dent Res 1993;72(6):1050–4.

[16] Antonucci JM, Dickens SH, Fowler BO, et al. Chemistry of silanes: interfaces in dental polymers and composites. J Res Natl Inst Stand Technol 2005;110(5):541–58.

[17] Friedman MJ. Porcelain veneer restorations: a clinician's opinion about a disturbing trend. J Esthet Restor Dent 2001;13(5):318–27.

[18] Van Meerbeek B, Peumans M, Gladys S, et al. Three-year clinical effectiveness of four total-etch dentinal adhesive systems in cervical lesions. Quintessence Int 1996;27:775–84.

[19] Van Meerbeek B, Perdigao J, Lambrechts P, et al. The clinical performance of adhesives. J Dent 1998;26:1–20.

[20] Magne P, Douglas WH. Porcelain veneers: dentin bonding optimization and biomimetic recovery of the crown. Int J Prosthodont 1999;12:111–21.

[21] Swift JR, Friedman MJ. Critical appraisal: porcelain veneer outcomes, part II. J Esthet Restor Dent 2006;18(2):110–3.

[22] Peumans M, Kanumilli P, De Munck J, et al. Clinical effectiveness of contemporary adhesives: a systematic review of current clinical trials. Dent Mater 2005;21(9):864–81.

ELSEVIER
SAUNDERS

THE DENTAL
CLINICS
OF NORTH AMERICA

Dent Clin N Am 51 (2007) 419–431

Porcelain Laminate Veneers: Minimal Tooth Preparation by Design

Galip Gürel, MSc

Tesvikiye cad. No. 143, Bayer apt. Kat 6, Nisantasi, Istanbul 34367, Turkey

A porcelain laminate veneer is one of the most conservative and aesthetic techniques that we can apply when restoring the human dentition. Since their development 25 years ago, interpreting the indications and applying the correct techniques has been key to providing their longevity [1]. Long-term (15- and 20-year) retrospective studies indicated that the success rates of veneers are as high as 94% to 95% percent [2,3]. Tooth preparation is one of the most important considerations in this technique. Bonding to enamel rather than dentin provides the best/strongest bond values when we want to bond porcelain to tooth structure [4–6]. When a porcelain veneer restoration is bordered on all margins by enamel, microleakage or debonding of these restorations is not likely to occur. A main objective of any restorative case involving these restorations is to keep the preparation simple and be conservative in reduction of sound tooth structure.

Many other considerations come into play as the preparation becomes more aggressive and dentin is involved. A rigid veneer behaves differently when bonded to a rigid surface, such as porcelain, versus a less rigid surface, such as dentin, and the composite cement can only absorb so much of the stresses to which the restoration may be exposed. To minimize effects and possible problems, we should be precise and careful about case selection and tooth preparation [7]. What if the teeth to be treated are not properly aligned? One of the major indications for using porcelain laminate veneer is space management. We are often asked to deal with spaced dentitions, crowded teeth, or a combination of both. The main challenges in these cases are visualizing the aesthetic outcome and providing the best tooth preparation to the ceramist to allow for the best aesthetic result.

E-mail address: galipgurel@galipgurel.com

0011-8532/07/$ - see front matter © 2007 Elsevier Inc. All rights reserved.
doi:10.1016/j.cden.2007.03.007

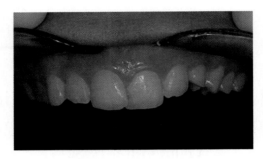

Fig. 1. An unaesthetic smile. The maxillary anterior teeth exhibit relatively dark color, short crowns, uneven gingival zeniths, crowded incisors, an uneven incisal silhouette, and a deciduous canine in the upper left quadrant.

Analyzing the smile

To have a solid understanding about the visualization of the final outcome, the existing smile should be analyzed carefully from a three-dimensional aspect.

Facial view

When the smile is analyzed from a facial view, we can only deal with the mesial-distal or vertical problems observed. In this particular case we see that the centrals are overlapping, which causes a vertical canting of the midline that is obvious even to the lay population. The existing teeth are short for this face proportion, and the gingival zeniths are asymmetrical (Fig. 1).

Viewing the teeth at a 45° angle (checking buccal-lingual dimension)

This view provides the opportunity to check the crowding more accurately. In this case we can see that the mesial-incisal tip of #8 is more buccally placed relative to tooth #9 (Fig. 2). In this initial evaluation, it is

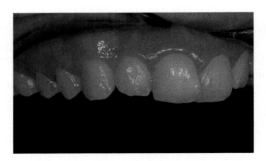

Fig. 2. Analyzing the smile at a slight angle allows for easy visualization of overlapping central incisors.

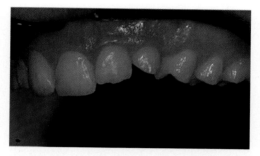

Fig. 3. The upper left aesthetic occlusal plane exhibits a reverse curve to what we would like.

difficult to decide which incisal edge position can be used as a reference point in a buccal-lingual dimension. Should we build up tooth #9 buccally or bring tooth #8 lingually?

Aesthetic occlusal plane

The third dimension to be checked in our aesthetic evaluation is the aesthetic occlusal plane. This evaluation can be accomplished by looking at right and left proximal views. In this case, a deciduous canine creates a problem related to aesthetic occlusal plane. This canine is too short in regards to the aesthetic occlusal plane (Fig. 3). The angulation of the centrals is preferred to be perpendicular to the aesthetic occlusal plane.

Functional evaluation

Functional evaluation of the teeth to bear the proposed restorations must be done carefully if we are to provide long-lasting restorations. One must be careful in checking the root of deciduous tooth #63 (European upper left

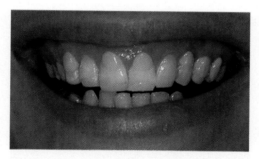

Fig. 4. Our first step is to align the incisal edges with a composite mock-up. The incisal edge position is ideally fixed with this mock-up. Additional composite is applied over the soft tissues to determine where the soft tissue gingival zenith should be after the periodontal intervention. The length-to-width ratio of the teeth is carefully planned out.

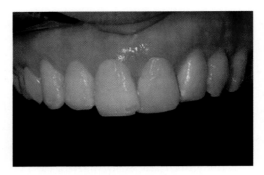

Fig. 5. After periodontal surgery (2–3 weeks of healing), a new mock-up is accomplished over the teeth to establish new proportions and relations to allow for an even better appearance of the patient.

deciduous canine) in the #11 position. If on the radiograph it is obvious that this deciduous tooth will most likely be able to withstand the lateral forces during occlusion, then a canine-guided occlusion can be planned. If there is some doubt, then splinting crowns using the deciduous canines in the #11 and #12 positions may be a good alternative.

Treatment planning

It is almost impossible to visualize the final outcome of this case using only an intraoral examination. The practitioner may begin to visualize and realize the aesthetic final outcome and share this information with the patient with the help of a composite mock-up [8–10].

Mock-up

Simply stated, a freehand carved composite can help the patient and the doctor visualize what the final outcome may look like. At this time the composite mock-up need not be as precise as a laboratory wax model (Fig. 4). It should give a general length of these teeth, the location of the facial

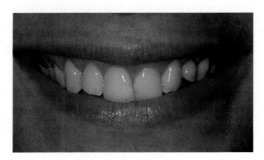

Fig. 6. Note the bleached teeth appearance.

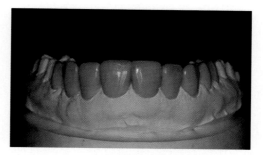

Fig. 7. The final laboratory wax model.

bulkiness, and its effects on the lip structure, phonetics, and occlusion [11–13]. This mock-up can be a great tool or guide if provided to the laboratory technician in a poured cast so that he or she may provide a wax model with a much more accurate idea of the possible outcome of the case [14].

More difficult cases may require a second intraoral composite mock-up. An example might be a case in which we need to alter the gingival levels, which changes the length of the restoration apically. It is often necessary for the dentist to make a second mock-up. After the periodontal surgery is performed and the tissue has healed, a new mock-up is produced (Fig. 5) to show new proportions and the new smile design.

This second postsurgical mock-up helps the dentist and ceramist to create precise teeth proportions relative to where the new gingival margins are positioned. In this case, a new impression is made out of the second mock-up and sent to the ceramist to provide guidance with the final wax model. A decision was made in this case to prepare the deciduous canine in position #11 and tooth #12 for crowns. They eventually will be splinted for better support and would provide group function design of the final wax model.

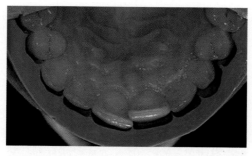

Fig. 8. This laboratory-fabricated silicone index can be used during the preparation to more easily reduce the teeth conservatively. Note that the silicone index cannot be seated on the arch passively because of the protruded position of the mesioincisal corner of tooth #8.

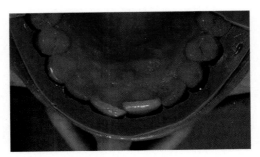

Fig. 9. In this case, aesthetic pre-recontouring is needed. The protruding surfaces of teeth were positioned labially, relative to the final contours of the finished silicone index. They must be trimmed back until the silicone index can be seated passively over the dental arch. Note the trimmed mesioincisal edge of tooth #8 and how passively the index is seated on the arch. After the aesthetic pre-recontouring. To test the final outcome of the proposed smile design, the aesthetic pre-evaluative temporaries must be constructed.

While the gingival tissue is healing from the periodontal surgery, it is possible to bleach certain areas with either an at-home or same-day bleaching method (Fig. 6). It is easy to visualize that the incisal mesial corner of #8 must be positioned and restored lingually. The best choice of treatment would be orthodontically moving it lingually and continuing with minimally invasive techniques. Time limitation for this specific case did not allow for this treatment option, however. This information is communicated to the laboratory so that the technician knows to trim the corner of tooth #8 slightly inwards when creating the wax model.

Laboratory communication

Two impressions of the patient's dental arches should be sent to the laboratory. One is the original existing tooth structure with all the diastemata and malaligned teeth (the initial study cast). The second one is the

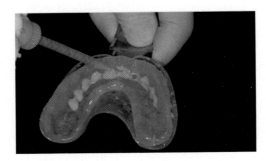

Fig. 10. An impression made out of the wax model is filled with a flowable composite (or any material of choice).

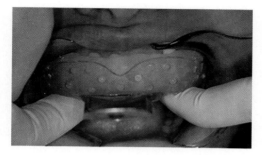

Fig. 11. An impression filled with a flowable composite is placed over the still unprepared teeth.

impression of the carefully constructed intraoral composite mock-up. The laboratory technician can examine the two casts and, using a silicone index, can finalize the wax model with all the details, as if building up the porcelain restorations. The technician is free to make a reduction on the facial surface of the protruding teeth (in this case, tooth # 8) and then finish the wax model according to the guidelines of our intraoral mock-up (Fig. 7). The technician should return the final wax model and a silicone stent so that the latter can be placed by the dentist over the existing teeth to see exactly where preparation is needed.

Aesthetic pre-recontouring

During the next appointment when the patient comes to the clinic for the tooth preparation, the dentist should have the silicone index. This index is made from the wax model and indicates the final contours of the teeth. The index is placed over the dental arch to visualize the existing positions of teeth on the dental arch relative to the final outcome of the wax model and veneers (Fig. 8). One problem that can be seen at this stage is that

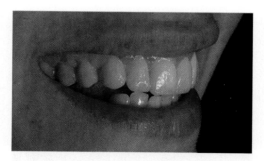

Fig. 12. The completed smile design, before any major tooth preparation is done with APT. This aesthetic pre-evaluated temporary construction mimics the exact final contours, texture, and shape of the final porcelain laminate veneers.

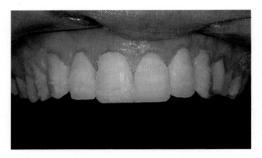

Fig. 13. This figure demonstrates the exact facial contours of the proposed smile design. Final tooth preparation can be done with the help of a silicone index right through the pretreatment temporaries, which gives the dentist and the ceramist the exact volume of reduction to allow for minimally invasive tooth preparation.

one or more teeth may touch or push the silicone index bucally, which indicates that these teeth are either rotated or positioned more labially than the expected final outcome. At this stage, those teeth must be trimmed down to place the silicone index passively on the dental arch. This process is called aesthetic pre-recontouring (APR) (Fig. 9) [15].

Aesthetic pre-evaluative temporaries

After pre-recontouring so that the silicone stent may fit on the unprepared teeth passively, a technique that allows for minimum tooth preparation can be performed. This technique calls for the dentist to use the laboratory wax model by taking an impression of this wax model and fabricating a transparent silicone impression. The dentist fills this impression with the flowable composite and places it over the unprepared teeth, light cures it, and takes the translucent impression material out of the mouth (Figs. 10 and 11). It would not have been possible had we rotated or bucally positioned the teeth. Thus is the importance of the APR because the transparent impression simply would not have fit on those teeth.

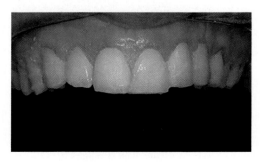

Fig. 14. Incisal reduction finished through the APT.

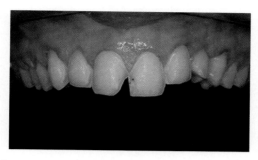

Fig. 15. Note that the mesioincisal corner of tooth #8 had to be reduced more than all the other teeth because of its protrusive position. All the other teeth are minimally prepared with almost all the enamel left on their surfaces.

After trimming the gingival margins, we have, for the most part, created an exact mock-up of final outcome of the case in composite attached to the patient's teeth. At this stage, because the patient has not yet received local anesthesia, we can evaluate the proposed aesthetic outcome (Fig. 12). The lip support of these restorations and the aesthetic length can be evaluated easily and should be approved by the patient. We also can evaluate the functional movements of the patient to see whether it would create an anterior constriction. The phonetics that otherwise may not have been able to be checked until after the final restorations are placed can be checked. This is a clear advantage in regard to allowing a patient a test run on what their restoration will look and feel like. Once this is approved by the patient, we can begin final tooth preparation.

This indirect/direct mock-up has been called APT (aesthetic pre-evaluative temporary) [15–17]. These provisionals can be double checked with a silicone index to ensure that they are placed in the mouth correctly.

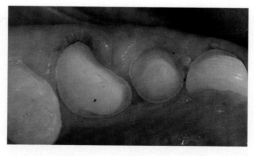

Fig. 16. The deciduous canine in the #11 position and premolar #12 are prepared to receive crowns connected to each other to support the functional loads they will be exposed to during lateral excursions. Note the 360° chamfer all around the gingival margin.

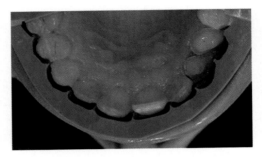

Fig. 17. The final check for preparation depth of the veneers and the crowns with the silicone index.

Tooth preparation through aesthetic provisional temporaries

The beauty of APTs, besides the evaluation of aesthetic functions and phonetic aspects, is that we have a great tool in our hands to prepare the teeth. We can use these APTs as a guideline to prepare the tooth structure. Because the APT resembles the exact final contours of the final outcome, such as the incisal edge position and the facial volume (contours) of the teeth, we can start preparing the teeth through the APT as if we were dealing with a simple case in which the teeth are aligned properly. We need not be concerned with how the teeth underneath are aligned (Figs. 13 and 14) [15]. If, for example, a tooth is too palatally placed (ie, more than 0.6 mm away from the facial contours of the APT), little or no preparation may be necessary. Generally, however, the only major reduction is accomplished with depth cutters followed by the round ended fissure burs. The clinician can proceed with the gingival margins and interproximal margins.

This case could have easily been overprepared had APTs not been used. Some studies have shown that on average, little incisal edge reduction is necessary, but often too much healthy tooth structure may be reduced in different preparations (Fig. 15) [18].

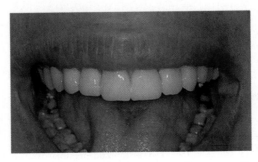

Fig. 18. After final impression, the provisional is temporarily cemented in the mouth, replicating exactly the final result to be achieved.

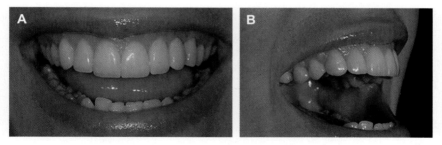

Fig. 19. (*A, B*) Final result in porcelain.

In porcelain laminate veneer preparation we tend to finish the gingival champher supragingivally unless we are dealing with severe discoloration or spaced dentition. After finishing the tooth preparation for the veneers, the deciduous canine in position #11 and first premolar tooth #12 were prepared for the ceramic crowns. They were connected to each other for the functional support and group function for the lateral excursions (Fig. 16).

Once the preparation is finished, the same silicone index is used to check and verify the correct preparation depths (Fig. 17). The final impression is taken, and the provisionals are fabricated. The provisionals are exactly the same as the APT. The patient has the opportunity to feel what the final restorations may be like during the week or two while the restorations are being fabricated (Fig. 18).

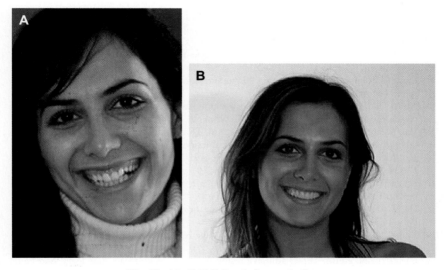

Fig. 20. (*A, B*) Full face before and after.

Laboratory procedures

In this case, a pressable porcelain was used with a layering technique. Whichever technique is used, the most important issue is that the ceramist use the same silicone index that was used to create the APT that was approved by the patient.

Summary

Porcelain laminate veneers have been one of the most used restorations for aesthetics. Although this approach is one of the most conservative treatment options, some rules must be followed. Aesthetics is a subject that is objective and necessitates excellent communication among the dentist, patient, and ceramist. The case must be carefully selected and treatment planned. The use of mock-ups, followed by a wax mock-up, APT, and silicone index not only lets us to get the best aesthetic, phonetic, and functional outcome but also allows for better communication with the patient and laboratory. Best of all, however, is that it allows for minimal preparation on the recipient tooth.

In addition to these techniques, the use of permanent diagnostic provisionals, which are worn for a short period of time while the restorations are being fabricated, could have a further impact on this solid communication. Patients have the chance to evaluate the aesthetics, function, and phonetics not only by themselves but also with their immediate circle of family or friends (Figs. 19 and 20).

References

[1] Calamia John R. Etched porcelain facial veneers: a new treatment modality. N Y J Dent 1983;255–9.
[2] Friedman MJ. A 15 year review of porcelain veneer failure: a clinician's observations. Compend Contin Educ Dent 1998;19:625–36.
[3] Calamia John R. Etched porcelain laminate restorations: a 20 year retrospective. Part 1. AACD Monograph 2004.
[4] Noack MJ, Roulet J-F. Rasterelelektronenmikroskopische beurteilung der atzwirkung verschiedener atzgele auf schmelz. Dtsch Zahnarztl Z 1987;42:953–9 [in German].
[5] Van Meerbeek B, Peumans M, Gladys S, et al. Three-year clinical effectiveness of four total-etch dentinal adhesive systems in cervical lesions. Quintessence Int 1996;27:775–84.
[6] Van Meerbeek B, Perdigao J, Lambrechts P, et al. The clinical performance of adhesives. J Dent 1998;26:1–20.
[7] Besler UC, Magne P, Magne M. Ceramic laminate veneers: continuous evolution of indications. J Esthet Dent 1997;9:197–207.
[8] Dietschi D. Free-hand composite resin restorations: a key to anterior aesthetics. Pract Periodontics Aesthet Dent 1995;7:15–25.
[9] Vanini L. Light and color in anterior composite restorations. Pract Periodontics Aesthet Dent 1996;8:673–82.
[10] Baratieri LN, editor. Direct adhesive restorations on fractured anterior teeth. Sao Paulo (Brazil): Quintessence; 1998. p. 135–205.

[11] Peumans M, Van Meerbeek B, Lambrechts P, et al. The influence of direct composite additions for the correction of tooth form and/or position on periodontal health: a retrospective study. J Periodontal 1998;69:422–7.

[12] Chiche GJ, Pinault A. Esthetics of anterior fixed prosthodontics. Carol Stream (IL): Quintessence Publishing; 1994. p. 33–52.

[13] Romano R, Bichacho N, Touati B, editors. The art of the smile. Carol Stream (IL): Quintessence Publishing; 2005. p. 7–24.

[14] Dawson PE. Evaluation, diagnosis and treatment of occlusal problems. 2nd edition. St. Louis (MO): Mosby; 1989. p. 274–97.

[15] Gurel G. The science and art of porcelain laminate veneers. Quintessence 2003;7:246.

[16] Gurel G. Predictable, precise and repeatable preparation for porcelain laminate veneers. Pract Proced Aesthet Dent 2003;15(1):17–24.

[17] Gurel G. Predictable tooth preparation for porcelain laminate veneers in complicated cases. Quintessence Journal of Dental Technology 2003;26:99–111.

[18] Castelnuovo J, Tjan AH, Phillips K, et al. Fracture load and mode of failure of ceramic veneers with different preparations. J Prosthet Dent 2000;83:171–80.

THE DENTAL
CLINICS
OF NORTH AMERICA

ELSEVIER
SAUNDERS

Dent Clin N Am 51 (2007) 433–451

Adhesion to Porcelain and Metal

Raymond L. Bertolotti, DDS, PhD*

*University of California, San Francisco School of Dentistry, Parnassus Avenue,
San Francisco, CA 94143, USA*

Advances in adhesion monomers and surface preparation techniques permit strong bonding of resins to metals and to porcelains. Most "pressed ceramics" bond in a manner similar to that of porcelains. The bond strengths to these materials can easily exceed the typical bond of resin to phosphoric-acid–etched enamel [1]. Using the strong bonds to these restorative materials, many innovations in tooth-conservative procedures are possible.

When we consider that tooth reduction correlates with need for subsequent endodontic treatment [2], the preferred treatment option often is one that relies on minimal tooth reduction. Adhesion, with less need for tooth reduction, is a highly desirable shift away from tooth preparation for mechanical retention.

This paper first presents some clinical examples where the use of adhesives clearly provides compelling advantages compared with mechanical retention and cementation. Then methods and materials to achieve resin adhesion to metal and porcelain are reviewed. Based on these methods and materials and the author's own clinical experience, specific adhesion protocols are given for some complex clinical applications.

The clinical advantages of using porcelain and metal adhesion

If we examine the cross section of a typical molar (Fig. 1), the distance from the occlusal surface to the pulp chamber is about 7 mm. A 3-mm occlusal reduction therefore leaves about 4 mm of remaining dentin thickness (Fig. 2). On the other hand, axial reduction of 2 mm leaves <1 mm of remaining dentin (Fig. 3). The 2-mm axial reduction is within current pressed ceramic manufacturers' instructions for tooth preparation.

Raymond L. Bertolotti owns stock in Danville Materials Inc.
* 188 Beechwood Drive, Oakland, CA 94618.
E-mail address: rbertolott@aol.com

0011-8532/07/$ - see front matter © 2007 Published by Elsevier Inc.
doi:10.1016/j.cden.2006.12.003
dental.theclinics.com

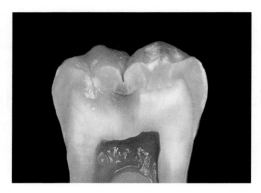

Fig. 1. Cross section of a molar.

With porcelain, metal, and even dentin adhesion equivalent to etched enamel adhesion, the obvious clinical application is the adhesion onlay. The onlay may be made of metal, porcelain, or pressed ceramic (Figs. 4 and 5). In these examples shown in Figs. 4 and 5, there is no intentionally cut retention form (Fig. 6). The "preparation" of the teeth was actually done by the patient through years of abrasion. No additional tooth modification was made before taking the final impression. Last photographed at 5 years and 3 months, this case remains successful after nearly 10 years.

While metal adhesion onlays have been successful for many years [3], clinicians have been reluctant to place occlusal porcelain onlays on molars. Presumably the reluctance results from reports of clinical failure of all porcelain molar crowns. However, a recent study [4], where 2 mm of pressed ceramic (Empress; Ivoclar/Vivadent, Schaan, Leichtenstein) was bonded to the occlusal surfaces of molars (partial onlays, not crowns), reported 100% success at 33 months. These onlays used 2 mm of pressed ceramic, like those demonstrated on the previous case. The high success rate is

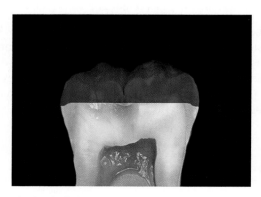

Fig. 2. Shaded area shows 3-mm occlusal reduction.

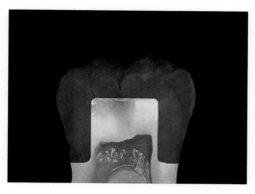

Fig. 3. Shaded area shows 3-mm occlusal reduction and 2-mm axial reduction.

presumed to be due to the ceramic being placed in compression during function, well supported by bonding to enamel and dentin.

Another tooth-conserving example is the cantilevered adhesion bridge (Figs. 7–9) of porcelain fused to metal, bonded to enamel. This is similar to the "Maryland bridge" but the "Yamashita adhesion bridge" uses resistance channels placed in enamel [5]. Such mesial and distal channels produce a highly successful result [6] when the metal is bonded to phosphoric-acid–etched enamel.

Porcelain veneers are a third compelling application of adhesives. The adherends are porcelain and enamel, porcelain and dentin, or porcelain and both enamel and dentin. Veneers can be done successfully with minimal intra-enamel tooth reduction [7]. The survival rate in most reports exceeds 90% at 10 years. The high success rates can be attributed to durable bonding and support for the porcelain provided by tooth structures (Figs. 10–13).

All the clinical examples illustrated above can generally be accomplished in a straightforward manner by following manufacturers' instructions for

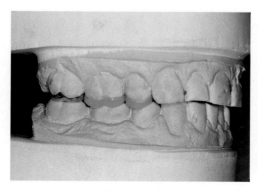

Fig. 4. Occlusal "adhesion onlays" of gold alloy and pressed ceramic.

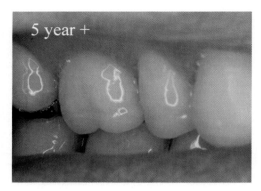

Fig. 5. Onlay 5 years and 3 months after completion.

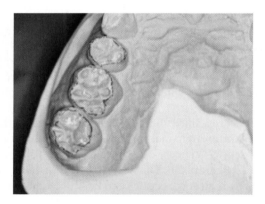

Fig. 6. Occlusal surface of cast with margins marked in red.

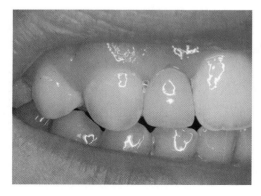

Fig. 7. Completed Yamashita adhesion bridge bonded to enamel.

ADHESION RETAINER

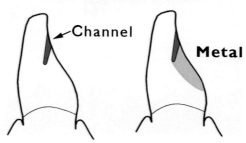

Fig. 8. Retainer preparation using intra-enamel channels.

the adhesive. While sometimes not as straightforward, porcelain repairs can also be highly successful. Some repairs require bonds to several dissimilar surfaces. After the discussion of metal adhesion and porcelain adhesion, some repair applications are illustrated and specific clinical protocols given for adhesion to multiple surfaces.

Metal adhesion

Mechanical retention

Adhesion to metal has long been a goal in dentistry. Resin-bonded "Rochette" [8] retainers were described in 1973. Retention was provided mechanically by composite resin locking into tapered perforations in the metal. A different approach to mechanical retention, using electrolytic etching to produce a microscopically retentive surface on the entire inner surface of the metal, was subsequently reported [9]. This etched metal is used for what is usually called the "Maryland bridge." Using the microscopic approach, two critical factors for successful adhesion to a metal substrate

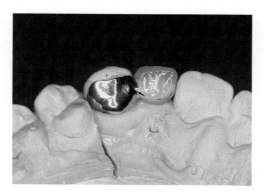

Fig. 9. Adhesion retainer on cast, lingual view.

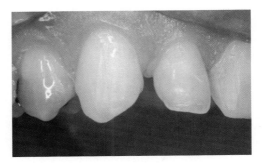

Fig. 10. Intra-enamel tooth preparations for a conventional veneer on the lateral incisor and "sectional" mesial veneer on the cuspid.

are (1) using an adhesive liquid with excellent wetting characteristics and (2) providing a high-energy metal surface to promote good wetting.

Substrate modification

Several researchers took a different approach to modifying the adherend metal surface. By itself or in conjunction with other procedures, sandblasting with aluminum oxide has become an almost universal procedure. Sandblasting with aluminum oxide can be done extraorally or intraorally. Sandblasting provides a fresh and uncontaminated surface that is high in surface energy and can be easily wetted by suitable metal bonding agents. Some other reported adherend modifications are high-temperature oxidation, immersion in an oxidizing agent, anodizing, and alloying the surface with a liquid gallium–tin alloy. In contemporary dental practices, these modifications do not appear to be used often. A different and more popular approach is adding a SiO_x–C coating by injecting a solution through a special flame [10]. Then a special silane is applied to the coated surface. This

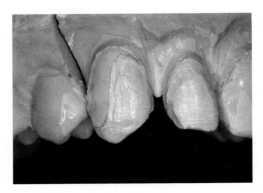

Fig. 11. Cast showing tooth preparations by marked margins.

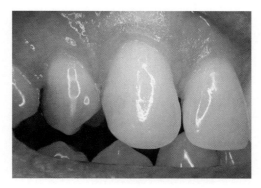

Fig. 12. Immediate result after veneers were bonded.

method is known as Silicoater (Heraeus Kulzer, Hanau, Germany). A more recent approach, widely used, is known commercially as Rocatec in the laboratory and CoJet chairside (3M ESPE AG, Seefeld, Germany). With this method, a tribochemical silica coating is sandblasted onto the metal surface to provide ultrafine mechanical retention. When treated with the silica-coating system, the surface is not only "abraded," but becomes embedded with a silica coating derived from silica-coated aluminum oxide particles. Metal and many other surfaces may be abraded with 30-μm grain size CoJet-Sand. Intraoral application is done with an intraoral sandblaster (Fig. 14), such as the Microetcher (Danville Materials, San Ramon, California). A specialized silane coupling agent is then applied.

Chemical modification of filled resins

Modification of the chemistry of resin to create affinity for metals is another approach taken to strongly adhere resins to metals. Following the development in 1978 of a new adhesive monomer, 4-META [11], a commercial

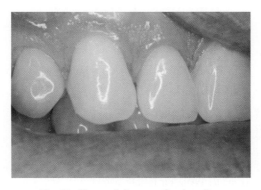

Fig. 13. Veneer 8.5 years after bonding.

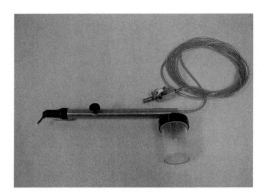

Fig. 14. Microetcher ERC II sandblaster with intraoral, contra-angle tip attached.

powder and liquid acryliclike product, Super Bond C&B (Sun Medical Co., Ltd., Kyoto City, Japan) was introduced in 1982 for adhesion to dental alloys and to tooth structures [12]. To improve mechanical properties of the adhesive resin and to change the handling characteristics, another approach was taken, which resulted in the product Panavia Ex (Kuraray, Osaka, Japan) [13]. It is a low-viscosity, quartz-filled composite resin containing a phosphate monomer known as M-10-P. Panavia is known to bond well to sandblasted base metals, but its bond to noble metals decreases when stored in water. To overcome this bond instability, the manufacturer developed a laboratory tin–plating apparatus, known as the Kura-Ace. It is used on noble metal alloys after sandblasting. Subsequently, two manufacturers produced portable tin platers capable of intraoral use [1]. These are Kura-Ace Mini (Kuraray) and Microtin (Danville Materials). A more recent product, similar to Panavia but using a different adhesion monomer, is Bistite II DC (Tokuyama, Tokyo, Japan). Tin plating has been challenged by the use of metal primers, presumably because metal primers are more expedient to

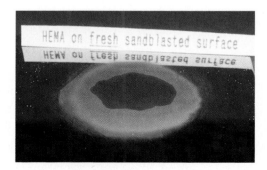

Fig. 15. Hydroxyethyl methacrylate on freshly sandblasted gold alloy surface. (*Courtesy of* Tom Blake, San Ramon, CA.)

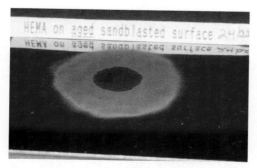

Fig. 16. Hydroxyethyl methacrylate on 24-hours–aged sandblasted gold alloy surface. (*Courtesy of* Tom Blake, San Ramon, CA.)

use. One recent study [14] compared the adhesive primers Alloy Primer (Kuraray), Metal Primer II (GC America, Alsip, Illinois), and Metaltite (Tokuyama) and the resin cements Bistite II (Tokuyama), Panavia F and Super-Bond C&B. All combinations appear to be potentially successful for the bonding of prosthodontic restorations, although there were reported differences in bond stability.

Unfilled "universal" bonding resins

As opposed to using a chemically modified filled resin, another method is to use a "universal" bonding agent, such as the All-Bond 2 System (Bisco, Inc., Schaumburg, Illinois), and then add a layer of filled resin. Primer B of the All Bond 2 System can function as a metal primer [15]. According to the manufacturer, when using the All-Bond 2 System, tin plating does not improve the bond strength of composite resin to sandblasted noble alloys. Similarly Clearfil (Kuraray) adhesives, such as Photo Bond and SE Bond, provide excellent metal bonding agents owing to the inclusion of the same adhesion monomer (M-10-P) as in Panavia.

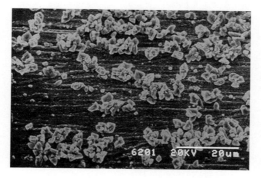

Fig. 17. Tin plate on sandpaper-treated gold alloy.

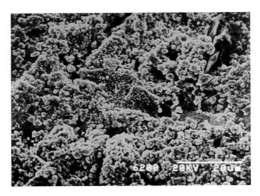

Fig. 18. Tin plate on gold alloy sandblasted with aluminum oxide.

Metal surface preparation

Contaminants on metal surfaces reduce surface energy and may compromise the bond strength to all resins. Sandblasting can remove such contaminants, creating a fresh, clean, and microscopically irregular surface with high surface energy. A high-energy surface is more wettable than a low-energy surface. An investigator, Tom Blake, looked at the effect of a delay after sandblasting, before the adhesive was applied. Blake, Director of Research at Danville Engineering, reported to the author in 2006 that the delay has a significant effect on wetting. Figs. 15 and 16 show the wetting of hydroxyethyl methacrylate (HEMA), a component of many bonding agents, at two elapsed times after sandblasting. When a measured drop of HEMA was applied to the "freshly" sandblasted gold alloy surface, a low contact angle and good wetting was observed. When the time was delayed for 24 hours after sandblasting, the HEMA did not wet as well, presumably because an absorbed layer on the metal surface lowered the surface energy.

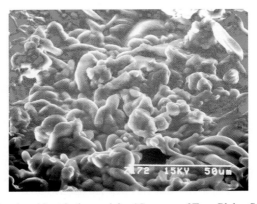

Fig. 19. Hydrofluoric-acid–etched porcelain. (*Courtesy of* Tom Blake, San Ramon, CA.)

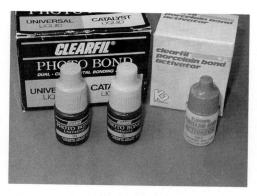

Fig. 20. Three components of Clearfil Porcelain Bond, which are mixed before use.

Clearly there is an advantage to having sandblast capability at chairside to freshly sandblast metals just before applying adhesive. It is common for dentists in North America to use such sandblasting. Outside North America, use is far lower but, according to the manufacturer of CoJet, many dentists worldwide use similar sandblasters to apply CoJet sand.

Sandblasting is generally used before tin plating of noble metals. In addition to providing added mechanical retention, the sandblasting activates the metal surface and makes it more receptive to tin plating. Somewhat analogous to the above HEMA wetting experiment is the tin plating activity on the sandblasted surface compared with a surface polished with fine abrasive paper. Plating tin onto an aluminum-oxide–sandblasted gold alloy surface results in tiny crystals covering the entire surface. In contrast, tin plating after abrasive paper treatment results in large crystals growing out of a few active spots. Therefore, it appears that the best tin plating results by electroplating a freshly sandblasted surface (Figs. 17 and 18).

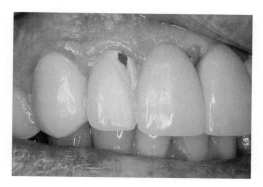

Fig. 21. Before repair.

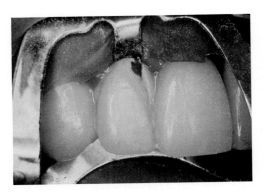

Fig. 22. Isolation.

The character of the tin crystal may play a role in the adhesion of resins to tin-plated metals. It may be that tin provides the enhanced mechanical retention or that a chemical bonding link to resin is established. In any event, the author's clinical experience with Panavia on tin-plated gold strongly suggests that the tin-plated metal-to-Panavia bond is superior to the Panavia-to-enamel bond. Debonds, although rare, invariably occur adhesively at the enamel-to-resin interface when Panavia is properly used. This observation is supported by shear bond testing [1]. It is interesting to note that "onlays" bonded with Panavia, when stressed to failure in a dislodgement test, broke the teeth cohesively rather than debond [13].

In summary, metal adhesion relies on an adhesive liquid with excellent wetting characteristics and a high-energy metal surface to promote good wetting. Modification of the adherend metal and modification of resin chemistry both play roles in achieving high bond strength and durability, important for clinical success.

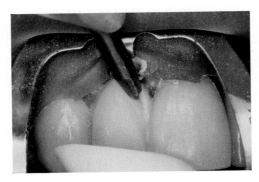

Fig. 23. Sandblasting of porcelain and metal with aluminum oxide.

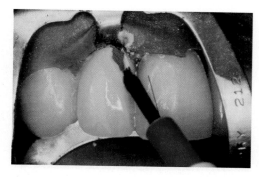

Fig. 24. Phosphoric acid cleansing of repair surface, followed by wash and dry.

Porcelain adhesion

Etchable porcelains and pressed ceramics

"Feldspathic" porcelain (eg, Ceramco 2; Dentsply, York, Pennsylvania) and pressed leucite– or lithium-disilicate–reinforced ceramics (eg, IPS Empress and Empress II; Ivoclar/Vivadent) are treated in similar ways before bonding. Being etchable with hydrofluoric acid and other fluorides (eg, acidulated phosphate fluoride and ammonium bifluoride), a strong resin bond can result from mechanical interlocking. Hydrofluoric acid (HF) solutions between 2.5% and 10% applied for 2 to 3 minutes are commonly used on porcelain and many pressed ceramics. The exact etching time depends on the substrate and the acid concentration. The glassy matrix of the porcelain is selectively removed and crystalline structures are exposed, creating a rough surface (Fig. 19). Some low-fusing porcelains and pressable ceramics do not etch well due to the low volume of acid-resistant crystalline structure.

Generally, etching is followed by application of a silane coupling agent. In addition to enhancing the wettability of the surface, the silane provides a chemical bond to the silica-based ceramic surface. Being bifunctional

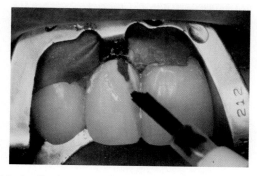

Fig. 25. Application of three-component Clearfil Porcelain Bond.

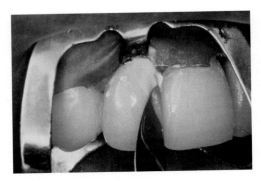

Fig. 26. Opaquer being applied, followed by light activation.

molecules, silanes bond to the silicon dioxide as well as copolymerize with the resins in the composite bonding agent that is subsequently applied. However clinical success has been reported [16] for bonding of etched porcelain veneers that had no silane applied. Presumably that success can be attributed to sufficient mechanical interlocking to resin created by etching of the porcelain surface.

Nonetchable ceramics

Nonetchable aluminum oxide or zirconium oxide surfaces (eg, Inceram; Vident, Brea, California) are not to be confused with HF-etchable porcelains. Since these oxides are not etchable with HF, they will not achieve a strong and stable bond by the same method as that used for porcelain [17]. Instead, certain adhesion monomers, such as M-10-P in Panavia, may be used to create a strong and stable bond. Likewise, Rocatec and Co-Jet are known to promote adhesion to these surfaces [17].

A little-known [18] product line called Clearfil (Kuraray) bonds silica-based ceramics without the need for HF etching; it only uses sandblasting.

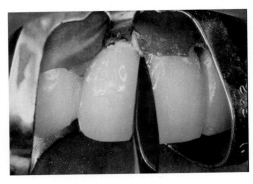

Fig. 27. Application of composite, followed by light activation and polishing.

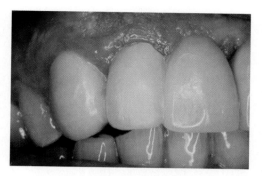

Fig. 28. Completed repair.

The porcelain bonds are equal to those achieved by HF etching followed by the best silanes [19]. Clearfil products are not the only ones capable of such porcelain bonds. However, unlike the other products, Clearfil products also simultaneously (with only one mix of material) bond to metals, etched enamel, and etched dentin. Clinical use of one of these products, Clearfil Photo Bond base and catalyst mixed with Clearfil Porcelain Bond Activator (Fig. 20), is illustrated later for simultaneous bonding to multiple substrates. This combination of three components is known as Clearfil Porcelain Bond. All Clearfil products are also capable of bonding to alumina and zirconia due to the Panavia monomer M-10-P in their formulas.

Complex clinical applications

Porcelain repair

Clinicians often face challenging cases where adhesion to multiple surfaces is required. Such a case is illustrated by the fractured porcelain on

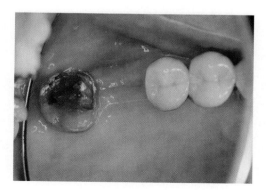

Fig. 29. Tooth loss, before replacement.

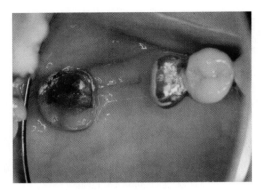

Fig. 30. Porcelain removed from distal abutment.

a five-unit fixed partial denture (Fig. 21). Successful repair with composite resin requires simultaneous adhesion to a base metal alloy and also to porcelain. Many similar situations also involve adjacent dentin and enamel (eg, an endodontic opening in a crown) where there would be metal, porcelain, dentin, and, perhaps, enamel. Illustrated below is a clinical example [1] where Clearfil Photo Bond (a sort of dual-cure "prime and bond") mixed with the Clearfil Porcelain Bond Activator is used to bond to all surfaces simultaneously (Figs. 22–28).

Pontic addition

Another challenging situation is the loss of a tooth adjacent to a relatively new three-unit fixed partial denture. With the capability for intraoral sandblasting and tin plating, the replacement of this lost tooth is easy. Porcelain is removed from the distal tooth of the existing restoration to create a preparation that will draw occlusally, in alignment with the preparation of the natural tooth distal abutment. A three-unit repair is prepared in the

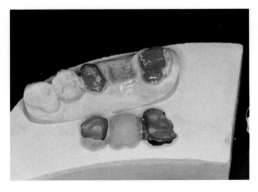

Fig. 31. Repair base metal casting with porcelain applied.

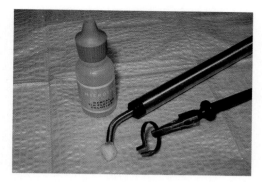

Fig. 32. Microtin plater with contact ring for intraoral connection.

laboratory. Since the existing metal is a noble alloy, sandblasting and intraoral tin plating is used to condition the prepared abutment. The repair casting only requires sandblasting since it is fabricated with a base metal alloy. The natural tooth abutment distal to the missing tooth is treated with self-etching ED Primer (Kuraray) before bonding with Panavia F. The Panavia F bonds to the ED Primer as well as to both conditioned metals (Figs. 29–34).

Other uses

Following techniques similar to those used in the aforementioned tooth replacement, a procedure for replacement of a missing acrylic facing on a gold-acrylic crown has been published [20]. Again, intraoral sandblasting and tin plating were used to condition the metal. Panavia was then used to bond a fully opaqued Artglass (Heraeus Kulzer) facing the conditioned metal. Using similar technology, modification of existing gold occlusals by intraoral bonding of new occlusal gold was reported [21].

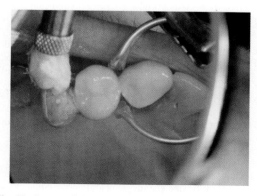

Fig. 33. Intraoral tin plating of sandblasted metal surface.

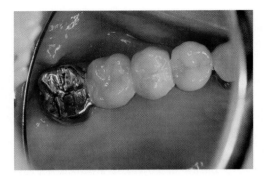

Fig. 34. Tooth replacement complete.

Summary

Development of adhesives and modification of adherends have made it possible to bond to metal and porcelain with enamel-like adhesion. Maximum tooth conservation is the compelling advantage in using these materials and methods.

References

[1] Bertolotti RL, Lacy AM, Watanabe LG. Adhesive monomers for porcelain repair. Int J Prosthodont 1989;2:483–9.
[2] Zollner A, Gaengler P. Pulp reactions to different preparation techniques on teeth exhibiting periodontal disease. J Oral Rehabil 2000;27:93–102.
[3] Uchiyama Y. Adhesion in prosthetic restorations. In: Gettleman L, Vrijhoef MMA, Uchiyama Y, editors. Adhesive prosthodontics. Chicago (IL): Academy of Dental Materials; 1986. p. 21–31.
[4] Guess PC, Stappert CF, Strub JR. Clinical study of press ceramic and cerec partial coverage restorations. Presented at the International Association for Dental Research 84th General Session. Brisbane, Australia, June 28–July 1, 2006. Abstract number 1639.
[5] Yamashita A, Yamani T. Adhesion bridge, background and clinical procedure. In: Gettleman L, Vrijhoef MMA, Uchiyama Y, editors. Adhesive prosthodontics. Chicago (IL): Academy of Dental Materials; 1986. p. 61–76.
[6] Botelho MG, Lai SCN, Ha WK, et al. Two-unit cantilevered resin-bonded fixed partial dentures—a retrospective, preliminary clinical investigation. Int J Prosthodont 2000;13:25–8.
[7] Freedman MJ. Porcelain veneer restorations: a clinician's opinion about a disturbing trend. J Esthet Restor Dent 2001;13:318–27.
[8] Rochette AL. Attachment of a splint to enamel of lower anterior teeth. J Prosthet Dent 1973; 37:28–31.
[9] Livaditis GL, Thompson VP. Etched castings: an improved retentive mechanism for resin-bonded retainers. J Prosthet Dent 1982;47:52–8.
[10] Vojvodic D, Predanic-Gasparac H, Brkic H, et al. The bond strength of polymers and metal surfaces using the 'silicoater' technique. J Oral Rehabil 1995;22:493–9.
[11] Takeyama M, Kashibuchi S, Nakabayashi N, et al. Studies on dental self-curing resins. Adhesion of PMMA with bovine enamel or dental alloys. Shika Rikogaku Zasshi 1978; 19(47):179–85 [in Japanese].

[12] Nakabayashi N, Takeyama M, Kojima K, et al. Studies on dental self-curing resins—adhesion of 4-META/MMA-TBB resin to pretreated dentine. Shika Rikogaku Zasshi 1982; 23(61):29–33 [in Japanese].

[13] Wada T. Development of a new adhesive material and its properties. In: Gettleman L, Vrijhoef MMA, Uchiyama Y, editors. Adhesive prosthodontics. Chicago (IL): Academy of Dental Materials; 1986. p. 9–19.

[14] Yoshida K, Kamada K, Sawase T, et al. Effect of three adhesive primers for a noble metal on the shear bond strengths of three resin cements. J Oral Rehabil 2001;28:14–9.

[15] Ciniome FA, Stojkovich L, Suh BI. Resin:metal adhesion and the all bond 2 system. Esthetic Dent Update 1993;4:38–47.

[16] Freedman MJ. A 15-year review of porcelain veneer failure: a clinicians observations. Compendium Cont Dental Educ Dent 1998;19:625–8, 630, 632.

[17] Kern M, Thompson VP. Bonding of glass infiltrated alumina ceramic: adhesive methods and their durability. J Prosthet Dent 1995;73:240–9.

[18] Bertolotti RL. Bonding to porcelain (forum). Practical Periodontics and Aesthetic Dentistry 2005;17:232.

[19] Llobell A, Nichols JI, Kois JC, et al. Fatigue span of porcelain repair systems. Int J Prosthodont 1992;5:205–13.

[20] Bertolotti RL, Miller D. Gold-acrylic facing replaced by intraoral bonding of a polyglass: a case report. Quintessence Int 1999;30:557–9.

[21] Bertolotti RL, DeLuca SS, DeLuca S. Intraoral metal adhesion utilized for occlusal rehabilitation. Quintessence Int 1994;25:525–9.

THE DENTAL
CLINICS
OF NORTH AMERICA

Dent Clin N Am 51 (2007) 453–471

Cements for Use in Esthetic Dentistry

Thiago A. Pegoraro, DDS[a],
Nelson R.F.A. da Silva, DDS, MSc, PhD[b],*,
Ricardo M. Carvalho, DDS, PhD[a]

[a]Department of Prosthodontics, Bauru School of Dentistry, University of São Paulo,
Bauru, Al. Otávio P. Brisola 9-75, São Paulo, Brazil
[b]Department of Prosthodontics, New York University College of Dentistry,
345 East 24th Street, Room 816, New York, NY, 10010, USA

Dental cements are designed to retain restorations, appliances, and posts and cores in a stable and, presumably, long-lasting position in the oral environment. Retention mechanisms for restorations secured by cements are reported to be chemical, mechanical (friction), and micromechanical (hybridized tissue). Retention of the restoration is usually achieved by a combination of two or three mechanisms depending on the nature of the cement and the substrate.

Acceptable clinical performance of dental cements requires that they have adequate resistance to dissolution in the oral environment, strong bond through mechanical interlocking and adhesion, high strength under tension, good manipulation properties such as acceptable working and setting times, and biologic acceptability for the substrate [1].

Many dental cements are commercially available, including resin-based and non–resin-based cements. Traditionally, zinc phosphate cement has been regarded as the most popular luting material despite its well-documented disadvantages, particularly, solubility and lack of adhesion [2]. Glass ionomer luting cements are also of great interest for clinicians, principally because these materials release fluoride that may prevent recurrent caries [1–3]. Resin-based cements are generally used for esthetic restorations (ceramic or resin based) and have become popular because they have addressed the disadvantages of solubility and lack of adhesion noted in previous

This work was supported in part by grants 300305/0-4 from CNPq, Brazil, and 04/12630-0 from FAPESP, Brazil.

* Corresponding author.
E-mail address: nrd1@nyu.edu (N.R.F.A. da Silva).

materials [1]. The advent of adhesive luting cements has considerably expanded the scope of fixed prosthodontics.

Restorative dentistry is constantly undergoing change, driven in part by new clinical applications of existing dental materials and the introduction of new materials. Currently, no commercially available luting cement is ideal for all situations. There has been considerable discussion on the properties and performance of these cements. Table 1 summarizes a variety of dental cements with their respective characteristics.

This article discusses the advantages and disadvantages of most common dental cements. Emphasis is given to resin-based cements for esthetic restorations owing to the large amount of discussion of these agents in the recent literature.

Zinc phosphate cements

Zinc phosphate cement has the widest range of applications in luting restorations, which includes the cementation of fixed cast alloys and porcelain restorations. It may also be used as a cavity liner or base to protect pulp from mechanical, thermal, and electrical stimuli [4]. The retention of restorations cemented by zinc phosphate materials (nonadhesive luting material) is largely dependent on the geometric form of the tooth preparation that limits the paths of displacement of the cast restoration.

Zinc phosphate cement can be regarded as the first "self-etch cement," because its acidity is capable of demineralizing the dentin surface and exposing collagen fibrils [5]; however, a traditional hybrid layer cannot be produced, because the acidic liquid segregates from the particles that are not capable of infiltrating the interfibrillar spaces. In fact, owing to the filtration phenomenon observed with these materials and concerns regarding possible hazard to the pulp, it has been recommended that dentin be covered with a layer of copal varnish before luting with zinc phosphate cement [4,6]. The adhesive potential of zinc phosphate cement was not appreciated in former usage in prosthodontics.

Because of its long-time use and excellent clinical performance, zinc phosphate cement has been regarded as the gold standard for comparative studies. If evidence-based dentistry is strictly followed, zinc phosphate cement has far more evidence of success than any other luting material available. Apart from this strong rationale for its use, disadvantages of the cement include the negative biologic effects (pulp irritation), the lack of antibacterial action, the lack of adhesion, and the elevated solubility in oral fluids [2]. Nevertheless, zinc phosphate cements continue to deliver successful results when used to retain metal crowns, porcelain-fused-to-metal crowns, bridges, cast posts, and other restorations. Even some all-ceramic restorations can be luted with zinc phosphate cements (eg, In-Ceram, Procera), but relevant long-term clinical data on their performance are still lacking.

Table 1
Current material classes of dental luting cements

Materials	Area of application	Strengths	Weaknesses
Zinc phosphate cement	Routine application in metal-supported crowns, bridges, and posts	Over 100 years of clinical experience	Occasional postoperative sensitivity Low hardness High solubility
Glass ionomer cement	Routine application in metal-supported crowns and bridges Limited application with high-strength ceramics during curing	20 Years of clinical experience Fluoride release Molecular bonding to the tooth substance Minimal dimensional change Simplicity of use Medium strength	Occasional postoperative sensitivity Sensitivity to water and mechanical loading
Resin-modified glass ionomer cement	Routine application in metal-supported crowns, bridges, and posts (esthetic) Limited application with lab-manufactured composite works Limited application with high-strength ceramics	Good routine cement Good routine cement Fluoride release Medium strength Molecular bonding to the tooth structure Low solubility Less technique sensitive Little postoperative sensitivity	Moisture-sensitive powder Swelling Not indicated for most ceramics
Adhesive resin cement	All metal-based ceramics, lab-manufactured composite works and posts (esthetics)	Over 10 years of successful application High adhesion qualities with pretreatment High hardness Low solubility High mechanical properties Good esthetics	Difficulty of handling Requires use of separate primers or adhesives Too strong for certain applications No fluoride release Occasional postoperative sensitivity

Glass ionomer cements

Glass ionomer cements are commonly used for cementation of cast alloy and porcelain restorations. These cements exhibit several clinical advantages [7], including physicochemical bonding to tooth structures [7,8], long-term fluoride release, and low coefficients of thermal expansion [7,9]; however, their low mechanical strength compromises their use in high stress-bearing areas [7,10].

The major benefit of glass ionomer cements is their ability to adsorb permanently to the hydrophilic surfaces of oral hard tissues, offering the possibility of sealing margins developed at the tooth-material interfaces during restorative and luting procedures [11]. Improvements in the formulation of the original glass ionomer cements have led to the development of hybrid materials that contain varied amounts of resin monomers. If the material can set properly by the acid-base reaction without the need of light activation, the material can be regarded as a resin-modified glass ionomer cement. Otherwise, if the setting mechanism is mainly directed by the light curing of the resin monomers, the material is more likely a polyacid-modified resin composite (compomer) and does not fit into the class of glass ionomer cements.

Resin-modified glass ionomer cements are indeed improved materials when compared with traditional glass ionomer cements. They represent the most used material among its class. The advantages of resin-modified glass ionomer cements include a dual-curing mode (light activated and self-curing), fluoride release from the cement, and higher flexural strengths in comparison with conventional glass ionomer cements. They are also easer to handle, including the fact that they are capable of bonding to composite materials. Although widely used as dental cements, glass ionomer cements have some disadvantages. One problem is that they do not always promote sufficient bond strength to enamel and dentin [12]. The other disadvantage is their ability to absorb water from the surrounding environment. Premature exposure to water leads to leaching of ions and swelling and weakening of the cement, whereas loss of water leads to shrinkage and cracking of the cement [13]. In general, bond strengths are greater to enamel than to dentin, leading to the conclusion that bonding occurs to the mineral phase of the tooth via chelation of calcium ions at the surface of the hydroxyapatite [14].

Glass ionomers remain the only materials that are self-adhesive to the tooth tissue without any surface pretreatment. Nevertheless, pretreatment with a weak polyalkenoic acid conditioner has been demonstrated to significantly improve their bonding and sealing efficiency [15–17]. The additional conditioning step becomes more important when coarse cutting diamonds are used and consequently thicker smear layers are produced. The increase in bonding efficiency must be attributed in part to a "cleaning effect" in which loose cutting debris is removed and to a partial "demineralization" effect in which the surface area is increased and microporosities for micromechanical interlocking or hybridization are exposed. More recently, chemical adhesion to partially demineralized dentin has been demonstrated [15–17] that favors the stability of the bond. In this respect, glass ionomers can be considered as adhering to tooth tissue through a self-etch approach [15–18]. The basic difference with the resin-based self-etch approach is that glass ionomers are self-etching through the use of a relatively high molecular weight polycarboxyl-based polymer, whereas resin-based self-etch adhesives make use of acidic low molecular weight monomers [18].

Glass ionomer cements exhibit properties beyond bonding to tooth structure. They can potentially be used as matrices for the slow release of active species, as has been previously documented for fluoride ions. They are able to bond chemically to surface active glasses, which have in their compositions substances such as calcium, sodium, phosphorus, and silicon. The combination of glass ionomer cements with these bioactive glasses (BioGlass or BAG) results in glass ionomer cements with surface activity properties [19]. The bioactive nature of BioGlass and glass ceramics is related to their ability to form a bonelike apatite layer on their surfaces in the body environment [20]. Some findings suggest that BioGlass could be used for remineralizing damaged dentin, and that it has potential as a filler component in mineralizing restorative materials such as glass ionomer cements [21].

A recent study [19] demonstrated that resin-modified glass ionomer cements containing BioGlass have the potential to mineralize dentin. In contact with saliva, these materials promote calcium phosphate precipitation on the dentin surface. The ability of these materials to precipitate minerals on the dentin surface may makes them promising resources for the treatment of dentinal hypersensitivity and for lining deep cavities in dentin.

Chlorhexidine is another example of a substance that can be incorporated into glass ionomer cements. Chlorhexidine can subsequently be released, resulting in the antibacterial properties of the cement. Additionally, chlorhexidine-releasing materials may be somewhat beneficial in preventing the action of host-derived matrix metalloproteinases in the degradation of exposed collagen [22,23]; however, the addition of chlorhexidine to glass ionomer cement may alter its properties. A recent study showed that the incorporation of chlorhexidine in glass ionomer cement resulted in increases in the working and setting times and a decrease in compressive strength [24]. Additional studies are evaluating the benefits of incorporating active substances and fillers in the basic formula of glass ionomer cements. Clinicians may expect several improvements in glass ionomer cement–based materials in the near future. For a more complete update, readers are advised to review the September 2006 issue (volume 34, issue 8) of the *Journal of Dentistry*, which carries the proceedings of the Second European Glass-Ionomer Conference held in May of 2004.

Table 2
Varieties of adhesive resin cements

Product	Company (location)	Bonding system per manufacturer	Indications	Curing mode	Additional features
Bistite II DC	Tokuyama (Tokyo, Japan)	Primer 1A+1B + Primer 2	A, I, and M	Dual-curing system	Different shades Metal primer
BisCem	Bisco (Schaumburg, Illinois)	Self-adhesive	A, B, I, M, and P	Dual-curing system	Fluoride releasing Auto-mixing syringe
Calibra	Dentsply/Caulk (Milford, Maine)	Prime & Bond NT	A, B, I, M, P, and V	Dual-curing system	Different shades Fluoride releasing
C&B Cement	Bisco (Schaumburg, Illinois)	All-Bond 2 One-Step	A, B, I, M, and P	Self-curing system	Dual-syringe mixer Fluoride release
Cement-Post	Angelus (Londrina, PR, Brazil)	Angelus Primer + Angelus Adhesive	A, B, M, and P	Self-curing system	Angelus silane
Choice	Bisco (Schaumburg, Illinois)	All-Bond One-Step	A, B, M, and V	Dual-curing system	Different shades Try-in paste
Duo-Link	Bisco (Schaumburg, Illinois)	All-Bond 2 One-Step/Plus	A, I, and P	Dual-curing system	Dual-syringe mixer
Illusion	Bisco (Schaumburg, Illinois)	One-Step	A, B, I, M, P, and V	Dual-curing system	Color modifier paste Try-in paste Viscosity modifier
Multilink	Ivoclar Vivadent (Schaan, Liechtenstein)	Primer A + B	A, B, I, M, and P	Self-curing system	Multilink Automix
Nexus 2	Kerr (Orange, California)	OptiBond Solo Plus	A, B, I, M, P, and V	Dual-curing system	Different shades Fluoride releasing Try-in paste Dual syringe

Product	Manufacturer	System	Indications	Curing	Comments
Panavia F 2.0	Kuraray (Okayama, Japan)	ED Primer	A, B, I, and M	Dual-curing system	Fluoride releasing; Different shades; Light shade especially for veneers
RelyX ARC	3M ESPE (St. Paul, Minnesota)	Adper Single Bond	A, B, I, M, and P	Dual-curing system	Clicker Dispenser RelyX; Veneer-exclusive veneer indication
RelyX UNICEM	3M ESPE (St. Paul, Minnesota)	Self-adhesive	A, B, I, M, and P	Dual-curing system	Activator/applier combination pack; Capsule mixing unit (for use with capsules)
Super-Bond C&B	Sun Medical (Moriyama, Japan)	Monomer + catalyst V + polymer powder	A, B, I, M, P, and V	Self-curing system	Different shades; Super-Bond C&B Quick Monomer; V-PRIMER concurrently for precious metal alloys; Porcelain Liner M concurrently for porcelain
Variolink II	Ivoclar Vivadent (Schaan, Liechtenstein)	Excite adhesive system	A and I	Dual-curing system	Different shades; Two degrees of viscosity; Try-in paste; Variolink II Veneer-exclusive veneer indication

Abbreviations: A, all-ceramic crown-inlay/onlay; B, bridge; I, indirect resin composite; M, metal; P, post and core; V, veneer.

Resin cements

Resin cements have become popular clinically owing to their ability to bond to both the tooth structure and restoration. The use of indirect restorations retained with adhesive procedures constitutes a substantial part of contemporary dental treatments. Metal and metal-free crowns, inlays, onlays, veneers, posts, and even resin-bonded fixed prostheses are now routinely bonded to tooth substrates by the use of adhesive resin cements (Table 2) [25]. The successful use of resin cements depends on several aspects related to the bonding mechanisms to both dental and restorative substrates. Recent publications have addressed many previously unknown issues that are key factors in determining the reliability of luting procedures with resin cements. These issues are discussed in the following sections.

Bonding to tooth structure: incompatibility issue

Except for glass ionomer cements and two self-etch resin cements available for clinicians (Unicem, 3M ESPE [St. Paul, Minnesota], and BisCem, Bisco [Schaumburg, Illinois]), all other resin cements require an adhesive agent to bond esthetic restorations to dental structures. The majority of adhesive systems used with resin cements are simplified systems because of clinical trends for reduced steps during adhesive procedures. These simplified adhesives are basically of two types: (1) etch and rinse single-bottle systems and (2) "all-in-one" self-etch adhesives. They are both somewhat acidic and hydrophilic in nature. During cementation, the acidic groups in the uncured layer of simplified adhesive agents (due to the presence of oxygen) compete with peroxides for aromatic tertiary amines of the luting agent, resulting in an acid-base reaction between the adhesive and the resin cement (Fig. 1A). This reaction minimizes appropriate co-polymerization

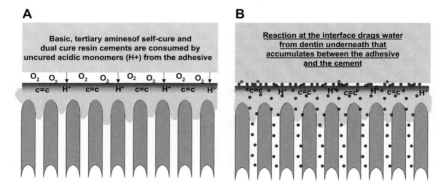

Fig. 1. (*A*) Basic tertiary amines of self-cure and dual-cure resin cements are consumed by uncured acidic monomers (H+) from the adhesive. (*B*) Reaction at the interface drags water from dentin underneath that accumulates between the adhesive and the cement.

between the two [26–28]. Additionally, the hydrophilic characteristic of such adhesive systems functions as a permeable membrane. This hydrophilic behavior permits the flux of water through the adhesive after polymerization [29,30]. The presence of water at the interface between the adhesive and the cement compromises the total bonded area and proper polymerization of the cement (Fig. 1B). Water droplets may accumulate at the interface and may function as stress raisers, leading to failure of the adhesive-cement interface [30]. This permeability problem could be partially solved by the application of an intermediate layer of a relatively more hydrophobic, nonacidic, low viscosity resin separating the acidic layer of adhesive from the composite resin cement [30,31]; however, this extra layer of adhesive may create a thick film, which would be a concern during the cementation procedure of esthetic restorations.

The water that accumulates at the interface derives from the hydrated dentin underneath (Fig. 1B). The negative effect of such water permeation on the bond strength of resin cements to dentin has been confirmed in in vitro studies [29,30]. These studies demonstrated improved bond strengths when the teeth were purposely dehydrated in ascending ethanol series before bonding. Because such dehydration of dentin is impossible to achieve in daily practice, clinicians are advised to use less permeable adhesive systems such as the three-step etch and rinse or two-step self-etch when bonding self- or dual-cured resin cements to dentin [30,31]. The major advantage of these systems is that they include a layer of a relatively more hydrophobic and nonacidic resin as the third or second step. This additional layer will not cause an adverse reaction with the basic amines of the cement and will reduce the permeability of the adhesive layer to water transudation from the dentin.

The incompatibility issue has brought up concerns for several clinical procedures. Practitioners should comprehend that unsuccessful treatment occurs owing to a combination of factors. First, permeability problems will not be in effect when esthetic restorations are cemented on metal, ceramic, or fiber-reinforced resin posts or cores. Moreover, problems when luting veneers with simplified adhesive systems should not be frequently experienced because clinicians typically use light-cured resin cements, and they are ideally bonded to enamel. The worst clinical scenario would occur when luting posts using simplified adhesives associated with dual-cured resin cements. Proper bonding to the apical portion might be severely compromised by the adverse interactions between adhesive and luting composite due to a lack of light exposure. Without light activation, dual-cure resin cements will actually function as exclusively self-cure cements. In this mode, the cement will take longer to cure, allowing more time for the adverse reaction and transudation of water from dentin to occur. Not surprisingly, some clinicians experience dislodgement of the recently luted post when they attempt to remove the provisional crown from a reconstructed preparation made with posts luted with resin cements (Fig. 2A–G). Based on

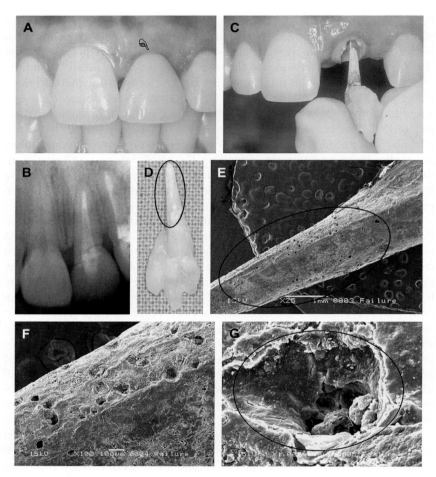

Fig. 2. Clinical case of dislodgement of luted post. (*A*) Clinical view of dislodgement of resin cement (Panavia) luted post (*black pointer*). (*B*) Radiographic view of the clinical case. (*C, D*) Closer view of the post dislodged. Note (*black circle*) the presence of resin cement on the post. (*E*) Scanning electron microscope image of the dislodged post. Note (*black circle*) the massive presence of bubbles, especially on the middle and apical thirds. (*F*) Closer view of (*E*), the presence of bubbles, which could be attributed to the water that migrated through the adhesive layer and to the poor polymerization that occurred, especially in the middle and apical thirds, denoting the so-called "emulsion polymerization." (*G*) Higher magnification of (*F*). The water droplets are kept trapped in the poorly polymerized cement (*black circle*), leading to degradation and crack spots along the adhesive-cement inferface. (*Courtesy of* Dr. Estevam A. Bonfante, Brazil.)

those limitations, some studies have suggested the development of a specific bonding system for this purpose [32,33]. Recent studies have shown that the push-out resistance of posts luted with resin cements was similar, regardless of the use of an adhesive system to bond to root dentin [32,33]. They have concluded that the retention of a post to a root canal is mainly determined by friction rather than by adhesive mechanisms. A truly adhesive luting procedure can only be achieved when clinicians combine the use of resin cements with three-step etch and rinse or two-step self-etch bonding systems.

Bonding to the surface of esthetic restorations (ceramics)

The ability of the combination of resin cement/adhesive system to adhere to dental ceramics depends on the microstructure of the esthetic restoration and the surface treatment applied [34]. Although roughening the surface by grinding or the application of airborne particles is considered a way for improved adhesion for most esthetic materials, silanization appears to be only effective for silica-based ceramics [35]. A durable and reliable bond for dental ceramics is usually attempted via two principal mechanisms—micromechanical attachment to porosities originated from hydrofluoric acid etching [36] with or without grit blasting—both associated with a silane coupling agent. Research evaluation of the bond strength between ceramic restorations and resin composite cements has resulted in varied conclusions as to the effect of varied surface treatments [36]. Controversy in the literature [36–39] focuses on the possible inefficacy of the silane coupling agent and operator's handling of the procedure.

Silane coupling agents are bi-functional molecules capable of bonding to the OH groups on ceramic surfaces and copolymerizing with the organic portion of the resin cement or adhesive. Silane primers contain a silane agent (usually γ-methacryloxypropyl-trimethoxy silane), a weak acid, and high amounts of solvents. To be effective, the silane agent must be hydrolized by the weak acid. Once hydrolyzed, silane primers have a limited shelf-life, and effectiveness progressively decays over time. The effectiveness of pre-hydrolized, single-bottle silane primers is unpredictable if the user is not aware of when the solution was activated. Clinically, the only indicator seems to be the appearance of the liquid. A clear solution is useful, whereas a milky-like solution should be discarded [35]. An alcoholic solution (one-bottle systems) stays transparent, and the signs of alterations cannot be identified; therefore, two-bottle solutions are preferred. Practitioners should strictly respect the expiration date and follow the manufacturer's recommendations for silane systems.

Understanding how the silanization process occurs on ceramic surfaces is of great importance to improve the effectiveness of silanes. When silane is applied to a ceramic surface and dried, three different structures are formed at what is called the interphase layer [40]. The outermost layer consists of small oligomers that can be washed away by organic solvents or water at room temperature [37]. Closer to the glass surface there is another layer of oligomers that is hydrolyzable. To avoid hydrolysis of this layer after cementation, which could compromise the coupling of the cement with the ceramic, some authorities recommend that it be removed with hot water before bonding to silanized ceramic [37,41]. Attached to the glass is a third layer, a monolayer, which is covalently bonded to the silica phase of the ceramic and is hydrolytically stable [37]. This remaining monolayer of silane is not removed by the previously mentioned procedures and is responsible for the actual bond between the ceramic and the adhesive/cement system.

Because it is not possible to clinically control the application of a monolayer of silane, undesirable excess must be removed before bonding. This removal can be achieved by several methods. One way is to apply the silane followed by hot air drying (50 $\pm$ 5°C) for 15 seconds for proper solvent evaporation. One then rinses with hot water (80°C) for 15 seconds followed by another hot air drying for 15 seconds [41]. This procedure eliminates water and solvent and washes away any unreacted silane (excess) primer components [41]. Alternatively, silane excess can be removed during the try-in step.

The try-in procedure is known to be a contaminant step; therefore, it has been recommended that it be performed before silanization. Clinicians generally perform the try-in step after receiving the surface-etched (hydrofluoric acid) ceramic restoration from a dental laboratory. Nevertheless, the hydrofluoric acid–treated ceramic surface is hydrophilic and more prone to be contaminated if the hydrophilic try-in paste is applied before the silanization step; therefore, ceramic surfaces should be silanized before the try-in procedure. Once properly silanized, the ceramic surface becomes hydrophobic, and the try-in paste can be removed easily by ultrasonic cleansing. Current scientific evidence [42] shows that if the try-in step is performed after silanization, bond strengths increase significantly. A possible explanation is the fact that the try-in procedure removes the excessive layers of silane from the ceramic surface [42]. Removal of this excess permits proper coupling of the resin cement with the monolayer silanized ceramic surface, improving the bond strength. Moreover, silane treatment alone seems to be effective to improve bond strengths to ceramic. When the try-in step is involved, it should be done after silanization, followed by ultrasonic cleansing for better bond strength.

Curing protocol for resin cements

Adhesive resin cements are available in light-cure, auto-cure, or dual-cure formulations, and their selection is based primarily on the intended use [43]. When comparing these cements, light-cure products offer the clinical advantages of extended working time, setting on demand, and improved color stability. Nevertheless, the use of light-cure cements is limited to situations such as cementing veneers or shallow inlays in which the thickness and color of the restoration do not affect the ability of the curing light to polymerize the cement [44,45].

Dual-cure resin cements are indicated when delivering restorations where material opacity may inhibit sufficient light energy from being transmitted to the cement [46]. In these situations, light intensity reaching the cement may be sufficient to begin the polymerization process, but an autopolymerizable catalyst is needed to ensure a maximal cure. Limited information has been published on the light-curing potential of dual-cure cements. Although early research suggested that the auto-cure system alone was not sufficient to achieve maximum cement hardening [47,48], recent literature indicates that the curing kinetics of dual-cure resin cements are more complex than previously thought. Some studies indicate that the light activating some dual-cure cements appears to interfere with the self-cure mechanism and restricts the cement from achieving its maximum mechanical properties [42].

Some dual-cure cements show their self-cure mechanism to be somehow limited when light activated in the dual-cure mode. This limitation may compromise the final mechanical properties of the resin cements [49,50]. One study [50] evaluated the degree of conversion (DC) of various resin cements at different cure circumstances. The Duolink (Bisco, Schaumburg, Illinois), RelyX ARC (3M ESPE, St. Paul, Minnesota), and Illusion (Bisco, Schaumburg, Illinois) resin cements cured well regardless of the activation mode (light cured, dual cured, or self-cured). These cements achieved maximum DC even in areas where the light could not reach. The Variolink (Ivoclar Vivadent, Schaan, Liechtenstein) and Choice (Bisco, Schaumburg, Illinois) cements showed similar DC when light cured or dual cured, but the DC was lower when those cements were allowed to self-cure alone, indicating that these cements would have their polymerization compromised and should be avoided in situations where the light cannot reach. Additionally, Calibra (Dentsply/Caulk, Milford, Maine) showed a poor DC when light activated in the dual-cure or sole light-cure mode. The maximum DC was obtained when the cement was allowed to self-cure alone. This information is of great importance for clinical practice because light activation of this cement is recommended by the manufacturer. Whether the same phenomenon occurs with other resin cements remains to be demonstrated. Although such information is not available for all resin cements on the market, it is advisable to delay light curing of dual-cure cements to the maximum time clinically possible. In this way, premature light activation will not interfere with the self-cure mechanism, and the cements requiring light activation for maximum DC will receive that energy after the waiting period.

Interestingly, alterations in the DC during different curing modes do not necessarily change the mechanical properties of the cements [50]. It seems that there is no linear relationship between the DC and the level of crosslink in the polymer network [51]. Nevertheless, cements that do not cure properly with light activation or that have a compromised self-cure mechanism may experience an adverse chemical reaction and permeability when associated with simplified adhesive systems. Clinically, this implies that the longer the resin cement takes to set, the greater the chance

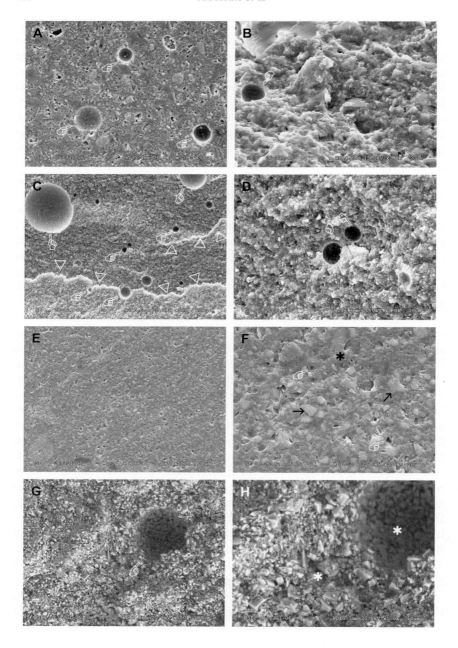

of adverse effects when coupling resin cements to simplified adhesives. Once again, these concerns could be reduced or even eliminated if clinicians used three-step etch and rinse or two-step self-etch adhesives.

Concerns regarding mixing and working time

Resin cements are often designed for specific applications rather than general uses. They are formulated to provide the handling characteristics required for particular applications. Figs. 3A–H show a series of scanning electron micrographs of different resin cements after mixing and subsequent polymerization. Entrapped voids due to mixing can be seen on polished or fractured regions of the set cement. Although entrapment of voids can be beneficial to reduce the shrinkage stresses generated at the thin cement layer [52], they can also function as stress raisers during tension or compression, generating crack propagation and, consequently, degradation of the cement interface. Voids are also observed in cements that use automatic mixing. Reduction of air bubble inclusion may be obtained with the use of resin cements that present an auto-mixing tip and deliver the mixed paste through a syringe-type tip directly on the surface.

The setting mechanism of dual-cure resin cements is usually based on a redox reaction of benzoyl peroxide with aromatic tertiary amines (represented by catalyst and base paste, respectively). One or both pastes contain a light-sensitive compound (camphorquinone) responsible for initiating the light-cure setting mechanism. After the pastes are mixed together and until light is activated, the adequate working time is controlled by inhibitors of the self-cure reaction or by the amount of peroxide and aromatic tertiary amines. Both the inhibitors and peroxides are organic chemical compounds susceptible to degradation upon storage; therefore, resin cements have a limited storage, and the setting mechanism of the cements may fluctuate during this time. In vitro evidence indicates that both the working time and setting time may be significantly altered upon storage, particularly if the storage temperature is far above that recommended (>18–22°C). Some cements present a shortened working time/setting time, whereas others present an extended working time/setting time [50]. This observation might be due to the instability of their components during storage time. Degradation of

Fig. 3. Scanning electron microscope images showing surface topographies of four different resin cements after mixing and curing. White pointers show entrapped bubbles due to mixing. (*A*) Polished surface (500× magnification) and (*B*) fracture area (2000× magnification) of Panavia F 2.0. (*C*) Fractured area of Variolink resin cement. Two fracture lines (*opened arrows*) occurring on the matrix and contouring entrapped bubbles. (*D*) Higher magnification (2000×) of entrapped bubbles. (*E, F*) Polished surface of RelyX ARC (500× and 2000× magnification). Filler particles (*black arrows*) adhered to resin matrix (*black asterisks*) are evident. (*G, H*) Magnification images (500× and 1000×) of RelyX Unicem. Huge amount of particles (*white asterisks*) without resin matrix in between can be seen even inside the enormous entrapped bubble.

peroxide would extend the working time/setting time, whereas degradation of inhibitors would shorten them. The implications of such changes on the mechanical properties of the resin cements are unknown; however, clinicians handling resin cements with a shortened working time may experience some clinical difficulties. On the other hand, increased adverse chemical reactions and permeability problems may be expected for resin cements with an extended working time and setting time.

Resin cement and water sorption phenomenon

When an all-ceramic crown is cemented into a patient's mouth, the assembly ceramic/cement/adhesive/tooth will be subjected to a watery environment. Resin composite cements should have not only low solubility and high color stability but also low water sorption because of esthetic and functional reasons [53]. The water sorption phenomenon has been demonstrated to have an important effect on the properties of composite resin cement after a long period of time [54,55]. This phenomenon diminishes significantly the flexural strength of resin composites. The reduction of flexural strength as well as modulus of elasticity [56] may be critical for thick areas of resin cement. Scientific evidence shows that absorbed water works as a plasticizer for the cements, creating unsupported areas underneath restorations and consequently increasing the chance of fracture of restorations under mastication forces. Clinicians should keep the cement film as thin as possible even in the inner aspect of esthetic restorations to minimize the consequences of the plasticizing phenomenon for resin cements [57]. The water sorption phenomenon of resin cements may also result in hygroscopic expansion [56,58] of the cement, but the influence of that hygroscopic expansion on the long-term durability of dental cements and, consequently, the esthetic restoration is not yet known.

Clinicians should be aware that cements that present an extended working time or setting time do not cure properly with light activation or have a compromised self-cure mechanism and will be affected by hygroscopic issues. Incomplete polymerization and nonconversion of monomer may result in loss of resin, and this may affect the biologic compatibility of the resin material [59]. Scientific evidence [60] has demonstrated that reducing the time for polymerization of light-cure cements to 75% of that recommend by the manufacturer may facilitate fluid uptake and dissolution of the resin, leading to staining and breakdown of the material resulting in failure of esthetic restorations. For that reason, maximum polymerization of the resin cement is crucial to minimize the water sorption phenomenon.

When using dual-cure cements, clinicians should delay the light-curing procedure to the maximum time clinically possible. In this way, the maximum degree of conversion of resin cement may be achieved after light activation, reducing the risk of excessive water uptake.

Acknowledgments

The authors thank the Department of Prosthodontics and the Department of Biomaterials of the New York University College of Dentistry. They are grateful to Dr. Byoung I. Suh for the knowledge offered in the description of the chemistry involved in the silanization process. The authors thank Dr. Estevam Bonfante for the generous gift of pictures (see Fig. 2A–G) included in this work. Hitachi S3500N SEM imaging (Fig. 3A–H) was made possible by the New York University College of Dentistry's cooperative agreement with the NIH/NIDCR.

References

[1] Meyer JM, Cattani-Lorente MA, Dupuis V. Compomers: between glass-ionomer cements and composites. Biomaterials 1998;19:529–39.

[2] O'Brien WJ. Dental materials and their selection. 3rd edition. Chicago: Quintessence; 2002.

[3] Diaz-Arnold AM, Vargas MA, Haselton DR. Current status of luting agents for fixed prosthodontics. J Prosthet Dent 1999;81:135–41.

[4] Brannstrom M, Nyborg H. Bacterial growth and pulpal changes under inlays cemented with zinc phosphate cement and Epoxylite CBA 9080. J Prosthet Dent 1974;31:556.

[5] Nakabayashi N, Pashley DH. Hybridization of dental hard tissues. Chicago: Quintessence; 1998.

[6] Brannstrom M, Nyborg H. Comparison of pulpal effect of two liners. Acta Odontol Scand 1969;27:443–51.

[7] Yiu CKY, Tay FR, King NM, et al. Interaction of glass-ionomer cements with moist dentin. J Dent Res 2004;83:283–9.

[8] Glasspoole EA, Erickson RL, Davidson CL. Effect of surface treatments on the bond strength of glass ionomers to enamel. Dent Mater 2002;8:454–62.

[9] Nassan MA, Watson TF. Conventional glass ionomers as posterior restorations: a status report for the American Journal of Dentistry. Am J Dent 1998;11:36–45.

[10] Kerby RE, Knobloch L. Strength characteristics of glass ionomer cements. Oper Dent 2002; 17:172–4.

[11] Mount GO, Makinson OF. Clinical characteristics of a glass ionomer cement. Br Dent J 1978;145:67–71.

[12] Mjor IA, Nordahl I, Tronstad L. Glass ionomer cements and dental pulp. Endod Dent Traumatol 1991;7:59–64.

[13] Wilson AD, McLean JW. Glass ionomer cements. Chicago: Quintessence; 1988.

[14] Wilson AD, Prosser HJ, Powis DM. Mechanism of adhesion of polyelectrolyte cements to hydroxyapatite. J Dent Res 1983;62:590–2.

[15] Inoue S, Abe Y, Yoshida Y, et al. Effects of conditioner on bond strength of glass-ionomer adhesive to dentin/enamel with and without smear layer interposition. Oper Dent 2004; 29(6):685–92.

[16] Inoue S, Van Meerbeek B, Abe Y, et al. Effect of remaining dentin thickness and the use of conditioner on micro-tensile bond strength of a glass-ionomer adhesive. Dent Mater 2001; 17(5):445–55.

[17] De Munck J, Van Meerbeek B, Yoshida Y, et al. Four-year water degradation of a resin-modified glass-ionomer adhesive bonded to dentin. Eur J Oral Sci 2004;112(1):73–83.

[18] Van Meerbeek B, Yoshida Y, Inoue S, et al. Glass-ionomer adhesion: the mechanisms at the interface [abstract]. J Dent 2006:615–7.

[19] Yli-Urpo H, Forsback AP, Väkiparta M, et al. Release of silica, calcium, phosphorus and fluoride from glass ionomer cement containing bioactive glass. J Biomater Appl 2004;19:5–20.

[20] Andersson OH, Karlsson KH, Kangasniemi K, et al. Model for physical properties and bioactivity of phosphate opal glasses. Glastechnische Berichte 1988;61:300–5.

[21] Yli-Urpo H, Lassila LVJ, Nä rhi TO, et al. Compressive strength and surface characterization of glass ionomer cements modified by particles of bioactive glass. Dent Mater 2005;21: 201–9.

[22] Pashley DH, Tay FR, Yiu C, et al. Collagen degradation by host-derived enzymes during aging. J Dent Res 2004;83:216–21.

[23] Hebling J, Pashley DH, Tjaderhane L, et al. Chlorhexidine arrests subclinical degradation of dentin hybrid layers in vivo. J Dent Res 2005;84:741–6.

[24] Palmer G, Jonesa FH, Billingtonb RW, et al. Chlorhexidine release from an experimental glass ionomer cement. Biomaterials 2004;25:5423–31.

[25] Peumans M, Van Meerbeck B, Lambrechts P, et al. Porcelain veneers: a review of the literature. J Dent 2000;28:163–77.

[26] Sanares AME, Itthagarun A, King NM, et al. Adverse surface interactions between one-bottle light-cured adhesives and chemical-cured composites. Dent Mater 2001;17:542–56.

[27] Cheong C, King NM, Pashley DH, et al. Incompatibility of self-etch adhesives with chemical/dual-cured composites: two-step vs one-step systems. Oper Dent 2003;28: 747–55.

[28] Suh BI, Feng L, Pashley DH, et al. Factors contributing to the incompatibility between simplified-step adhesives and chemically cured or dual-cured composites. Part III. Effect of acidic resin monomers. J Adhes Dent 2003;5:267–82.

[29] Tay FR, Pashley DH, Suh BI, et al. Single-step adhesives are permeable membranes. J Dent 2002;30:371–82.

[30] Carvalho RM, Pegoraro TA, Tay FR, et al. Adhesive permeability affects coupling of resin cements that utilise self-etching primers to dentin. J Dent 2004;32:55–65.

[31] King NM, Tay FR, Pashley DH, et al. Conversion of one-step to two-step self-etch adhesives for improved efficacy and extended application. Am J Dent 2005;18:126–34.

[32] Goracci C, Fabianelli A, Sadek FT, et al. The contribution of friction to the dislocation resistance of bonded fiber posts. J Endod 2005;31:608–12.

[33] Cury AH, Goracci C, de Lima Navarro MF, et al. Effect of hygroscopic expansion on the push-out resistance of glass ionomer-based cements used for the luting of glass fiber posts. J Endod 2006;32:537–40.

[34] Clelland NL, Warchol N, Kerby RE, et al. Influence of interface surface conditions on indentation failure of simulated bonded ceramic onlays. Dent Mater 2006;22 99–106.

[35] Blatz MB, Sadan A, Kern M. Resin-ceramic bonding: a review of the literature. J Prosthet Dent 2003;89:268–74.

[36] Calamia JR, SR. Effect of coupling agents on bond strength of etched porcelain [abstract 79]. J Denta Res 1984;63:179.

[37] Hooshmand T, van Noort R, Keshvad A. Bond durability of the resin-bonded and silane-treated ceramic surface. Dent Mater 2002;18(2):179–88.

[38] Barghi N, Chung K, Farshchian F, et al. Effects of the solvents on bond strength of resin bonded porcelain. J Oral Rehabil 1999;26:853–7.

[39] Roulet JF, Soderholm KJ, Longmate J. Effects of treatments and storage conditions on ceramic/composite bond strength. J Dent Res 1995;74:381–7.

[40] Ishida H. Structural gradient in the silane coupling agent layers and its influence on the mechanical and physical properties of composites. New York: Plenum Press; 1985. 25–50.

[41] Hooshmand T, van Noort R, Keshvad A. Storage effect of a pre-activated silane on the resin to ceramic bond. Dent Mater 2004;20:635–42.

[42] Carvalho RM, Manso AP, Pegoraro TA, Suh BI. Bonding aspects of luting resin cements. Trans Acad Dent Mater, in press.

[43] Platt JA. Resin cements: into the 21st century. Compendium of Continued Education in Dentistry 1999;20:1173–8.

[44] Caughman WF, Daniel ME, Chan CN, et al. Curing potential of dual-polymerizable resin cements in simulated clinical situations. J Prosthet Dent 2001;85:479–84.

[45] Breeding LC, Dixon DL, Caughman WF. The curing potential of light-activated composite resin luting agents. J Prosthet Dent 1991;65:512–8.

[46] Myers ML, Caughman WF, Rueggeberg FA. Effect of restoration composition, shade, and thickness on the cure of a photoactivated resin cement. J Prosthodont 1994;3:149–57.

[47] El-Badrawy WA, El-Mowafy OM. Chemical versus dual curing of resin inlay cements. J Prosthet Dent 1995;73:515–24.

[48] Hasegawa EA, Boyer DB, Chan DC. Hardening of dual-cured cements under composite resin inlays. J Prosthet Dent 1991;66:187–92.

[49] Velarde ME, Miller MB, Mariño KL, et al. Hardness of dual-cure resin cements using three polymerization methods. Available at: http://iadr.confex.com/iadr/2005Balt/techprogram/abstract_61904.htm.

[50] Sharp LJ, Yin R, Kang WH, et al. Comparison of curing of resin cements. Available at: http://iadr.confex.com/iadr/2005Balt/techprogram/abstract_60685.htm.

[51] Peutzfeldt A, Asmussen E. Investigations on polymer structure of dental resinous materials. Transaction of Academy of Dental Materials 2004;18:81–104.

[52] Carvalho RM, Pereira JC, Yoshiyama M, et al. A review of polymerization contraction: the influence of stress development versus stress relief. Oper Dent 1996;21(1):17–24.

[53] Tanoue N, Koishi Y, Atsuta M, et al. Properties of dual-curable luting composites polymerized with single and dual curing modes. J Oral Rehabil 2003;30(10):1015–21.

[54] Fan PL, Edahl A, Leung RL, et al. Alternative interpretations of water sorption values of composite resins. J Dent Res 1985;64(1):78–80.

[55] Ortengren U, Elgh U, Spasenoska V, et al. Water sorption and flexural properties of a composite resin cement. Int J Prosthodont 2000;13(2):141–7.

[56] Oysaed H, Ruyter IE. Composites for use in posterior teeth: mechanical properties tested under dry and wet conditions. J Biomed Mater Res 1986;20(2):261–71.

[57] Ferracane JL, Berge HX, Condon JR. In vitro aging of dental composites in water—effect of degree of conversion, filler volume, and filler/matrix coupling. J Biomed Mater Res 1998; 42(3):465–72.

[58] Huang M, Niu X, Shrotriya P, et al. Contact damage of dental multilayers: viscous deformation and fatigue mechanisms. Journal of Engineering Materials and Technology 2005; 127(33):33–9.

[59] Braden M, Clarke RL. Water absorption characteristics of dental microfine composite filling materials. Biomaterials 1994;5:369–72.

[60] Pearson GJ, Longman CM. Water sorption and solubility of resin-based materials following inadequate polymerization by a visible-light curing system. J Oral Rehabil 1989;16:57–60.

THE DENTAL
CLINICS
OF NORTH AMERICA

ELSEVIER
SAUNDERS

Dent Clin N Am 51 (2007) 473–485

Clinical Steps to Predictable Color Management in Aesthetic Restorative Dentistry

Stephen J. Chu, DMD, MSD, CDT

*Department of Periodontics and Implant Dentistry, New York University College of Dentistry,
345 East 24th Street, New York, NY 10010, USA*

The shade matching of a restoration is the critical final step in aesthetic restorative dentistry once morphology and occlusion are addressed. The variables in the dental treatment room and human error are recognized obstacles first divulged by Dr. Jack Preston at USC Dental School. Color is both a science and an art, and can often be difficult to measure.

Conventional shade methods and technology by itself have limitations, because technicians require more visual information to interpret shade information. Advances in technology have greatly elevated the likelihood of a clinically acceptable shade match through accurate shade analysis, if properly performed. After much research and clinical evaluation, this article addresses a culmination of knowledge that embodies how the author perceives predictable shade matching.

A step-by-step protocol to shade matching is comprehensively outlined through a case study using a combination of technology-based instrumentation, conventional techniques (ie, shade tabs), and reference photography: a wonderful way for predictable shade matching that, if performed properly, can limit costly remakes.

Predictable shade matching protocol

Step 1: evaluation

This phase of treatment may be the most clinically significant because proper shade matching is directly dependent on the tooth type (ie, whether the tooth is high or low in translucency) (Fig. 1).

E-mail address: schudmd@aol.com

0011-8532/07/$ - see front matter © 2007 Published by Elsevier Inc.
doi:10.1016/j.cden.2007.02.004

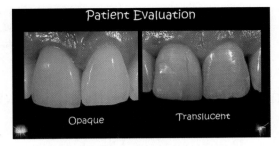

Fig. 1. The central incisor teeth represented in the photograph on the left are low in translucency and high in opacity. Note the lack of translucency throughout the tooth structure. Matching these teeth is best served with metal-ceramic restorations or computer aided design-computer aided manufacturing (CAD-CAM)–based ceramics. The central incisor teeth on the right are higher in translucency. Materials selection and restoration type for these teeth may comprise the following: all-ceramic refractory cast or platinum foil veneer or crown; leucite-reinforced pressable ceramics; or a porcelain butt margin CAD-CAM–based ceramic restoration, such as zirconia.

Preoperative evaluation affects material selection because the choices of materials that can be used for the definitive restoration (ie, metal-ceramic or high-strength computer aided design-computer aided manufacturing (CAD-CAM)–based ceramics, such as alumina or zirconia [Fig. 2]) ultimately dictate the tooth preparation design (Fig. 3). The stump shade of the tooth must be taken into consideration because it may influence the value, chroma, and hue of the final restoration if a translucent or semitranslucent material is used (Fig. 4).

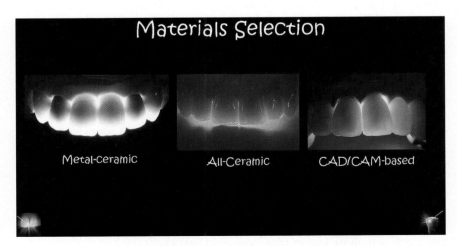

Fig. 2. High-strength CAD-CAM materials are available in various types of ceramic (ie, alumina and zirconia) to satisfy the strength and aesthetic requirements anywhere in the mouth. They possess light transmission qualities greater than that of metal-ceramic restorations. Optical properties vary; familiarity with these materials is a must because CAD-CAM has become increasingly popular and widely accepted among dentists and laboratory technicians alike.

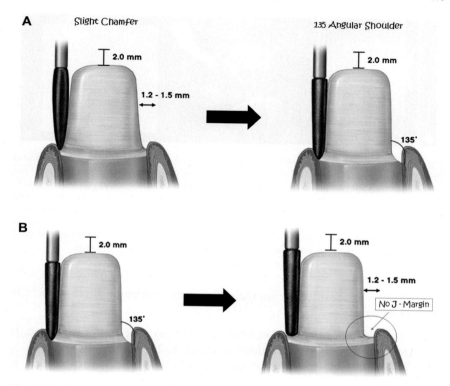

Fig. 3. Tooth preparation design may take many forms and is primarily dependent on the material chosen and collar design for the final restoration. A slight chamfer preparation (*left A*) requires a metal collar design because there is minimal reduction in the cervical one third of the tooth. With an angular shoulder (135-degree) preparation (*right A; left B*) or full rounded shoulder (*right B*), a zero metal collar or ceramic butt margin, respectively, can be selected because greater tooth is reduced in the gingival one third. CAD-CAM–based restorations or a pressed leucite-reinforced material can be selected with the equivalent preparation designs previously mentioned for the same reason.

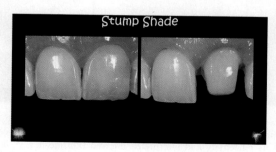

Fig. 4. The stump shade of the tooth must be taken into consideration because it may influence the value, chroma, and hue of the final restoration if a translucent or semi-translucent material is used.

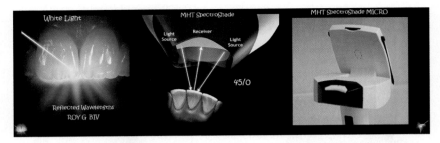

Fig. 5. Spectrophotometers measure and record the amount of visible radiant energy reflected by the teeth one wavelength at a time for each hue, value, and chroma present in the entire visible spectrum. It uses reflectance technology because it only calculates the quantity and quality of light that is not absorbed by the measured tooth. Present spectrophotometers used in dentistry illuminate the teeth at a 45-degree angle of incidence to the object to eliminate reflectance glare and thereby distortion of the image. The reflected light from the image is captured at a zero-degree angle of incidence. A specific and unique fingerprint of the image is then recorded at intervals of 10 nm throughout the whole visible light spectrum (400–800 nm).

Questions to consider during the preoperative patient evaluation include the following:

1. Is there significant variation of shade from gingival, to body, to incisal?
2. Are there any characterizations or effects in the tooth?
3. Can the patient's teeth be categorized as high in translucency or high in opacity?
4. Can materials selection affect the final aesthetic outcome of the restoration?

After those questions have been addressed a treatment plan can be developed, and the clinician can determine the ideal material selection and preparation for the restoration.

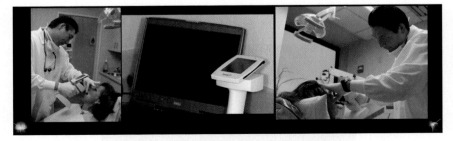

Fig. 6. Portable handheld spectrophotometers, such as the SpectroShade MICRO System from MHT, use dual digital cameras and LED light technology to measure the color of teeth and allow readings of its reflectivity and interpreted inferred translucency. A flip-up color PDA screen allows easy image visualization during image capture and immediate chair-side shade analysis without requiring the unit to interface with a computer.

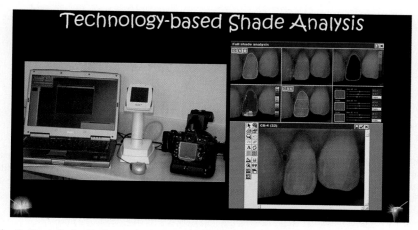

Fig. 7. Once the image is acquired, the teeth are analyzed for overall basic shade and the gingival-body-incisal shade. A composite shade analysis map including delta E values can be acquired once the shade information has been downloaded to the computer database using the SpectroShade software.

Step 2: image capture and shade analysis

One way to analyze the shade is to use technology (SpectroShade Micro, MHT S.P.A., Milan, Italy) (Fig. 5), because it is the least influenced by contrast effects and visual discrepancies associated with improper lighting. Technology requires image capture (Fig. 6) or image acquisition. Once the images are brought into the database and stored, they can then be analyzed for shade (Figs. 7 and 8). Today's technology streamlines shade analysis by indicating which shade tabs the clinician should select for reference photography (shade communication).

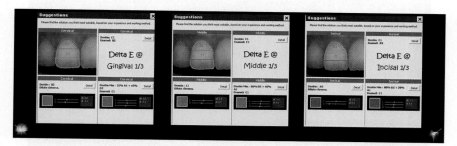

Fig. 8. Besides giving a gingival-body-incisal map of the tooth, delta E values can be generated and quantified. This is unique to spectrophotometers because they have true numerical values associated with the tooth shade and these numbers can be mathematically compared with the values of shade tabs. The change in E (delta E) can then be calculated. A delta E of 0 is a perfect match. The human eye is sensitive to a delta E of 2 in regards to value [L]; any number greater than 2 is noticeable and not a clinically acceptable match.

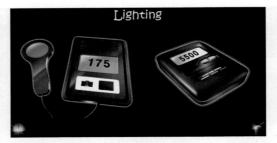

Fig. 9. A light meter can be used in the treatment room to assess the proper quantitative amount of foot-candle of light (175) illuminating the treatment room environment. In addition, a color temperature meter can be used to assess the quality of light, which should be at 5500–6500 K.

Conventional means of shade selection can also be used effectively. Shade tabs remain the most common tools used for conventional shade analysis. Care must be taken to create the proper lighting quantity (175 foot-candle of light) and quality (5500–6500 K) (Fig. 9) in the treatment room to control the environment under which shade is selected. This reduces the unhelpful variables that can negatively influence conventional shade analysis. In addition, laboratory special effect shade tabs can be used to select the special effect porcelain materials that are used in fabrication of the restoration (Fig. 10).

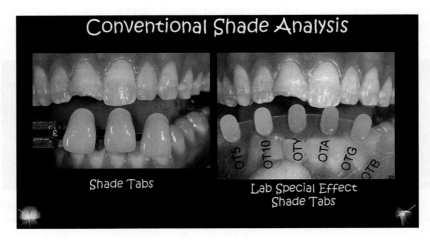

Fig. 10. Conventional shade guide tabs can be used effectively under proper controlled lighting and consistent exposure of digital photographs. Laboratory shade guide special effect tabs representing the ceramics used in fabrication can also be used clinically for shade.

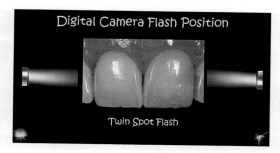

Fig. 11. Photographs of these central incisors with lighting from a twin spot flash from both sides.

Step 3: transferring the information into a visual format (shade communication)

High-quality digital photographs are the best means to communicate shade. With digital photography, images can be immediately evaluated and assessed for quality. With cost-efficient storage media devices, there is no penalty for taking a poor image because it can be erased. Special effects and characterizations can be best visualized by altering the object's exposure to brightness, viewing angle, and flash orientation (Figs. 11 and 12).

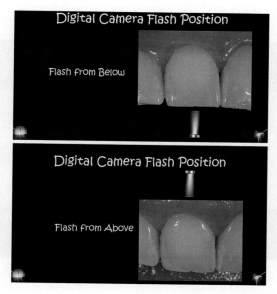

Fig. 12. Flash light emanating from below and from the top allows nuances in tooth shade and characterization to be clearly visualized. A lower exposure image should be provided to the technician, thereby allowing visualization of special effects and characterizations in the tooth shade.

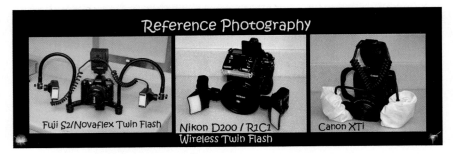

Fig. 13. A high-quality digital camera system is recommended for use because it produces qual-ity images for shade interpretation. Images can be downloaded onto a CF II/III or SD card. There is no penalty for a poor image taken because they can be evaluated immediately and erased if necessary. High-capacity storage media (CF or SD cards) allow literally hundreds of images to be taken before formatting and eliminating them from the card.

Shade tabs and reference photography should be used together to gather and communicate the precise shade information, respectively. Shade tabs provide a visual reference marker, and using contrasting shade tabs that are both bright and dark allows clinicians and their laboratory technicians to determine better the value and chroma of the restoration. Taking refer-ence photography provides the laboratory technician with a better under-standing of how the shade tabs compare with the shade of the surrounding dentition and the value changes of the tooth to be matched

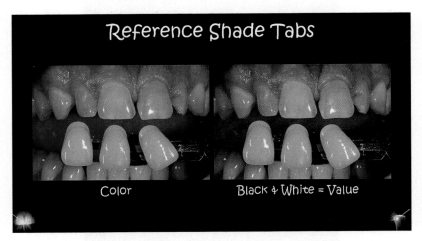

Fig. 14. Reference photographs using contrasting shade tabs that are both bright and dark, and the actual matched gingival-body-incisal tab, provide a better overall picture of the surrounding dentition and the tooth to be matched. The color photograph can be converted to a black and white image, which aids in assessing which value shade tab is the most significant variable. An 18% gray card background can be used to help limit visual distractions that can lead to poor shade perception.

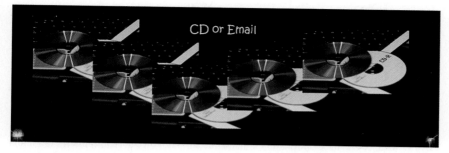

Fig. 15. E-mail allows for instant transferal of shade information to and from the laboratory provided the server allows high-capacity internet file transfer. The shade data may be mailed to the laboratory on a CD along with the actual case.

(Fig. 13). As an adjunct, black and white photographs are helpful in determining value, which is the most significant variable (Fig. 14).

Once the shade information is gathered by the clinician, it must be delivered to the laboratory. This can be accomplished by sending it as a hard copy stored on a CD, or by e-mail (Fig. 15). Reference photography and written descriptions are the most critical pieces of information for accurate shade communication that must be sent to the laboratory. By using technology, all of the analysis information can be delivered electronically.

Step 4: interpreting the shade information (interpretation)

When the laboratory technician receives the shade information, he or she must interpret all of the pieces of submitted information. A color map report alone is insufficient; all materials should be taken into account when interpreting the shade (Figs. 16 and 17). The reference photography is tantamount to the laboratory technician to understand better the shade tab

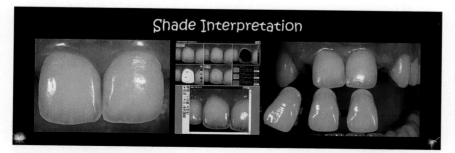

Fig. 16. Photographs of the tooth to be matched, digital shade reports, and reference photographs can be compiled as a composite collage to allow easy and simple shade interpretation and understanding of color. Interpretation of shade information can be termed "visual understanding" of the color.

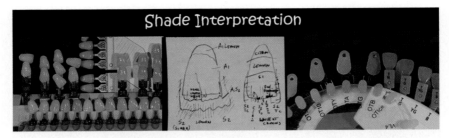

Fig. 17. With all the shade information at hand, the laboratory technician translates this information into the language of the ceramic system to be used.

selection and the variance in value and chroma. The digital color map provides a close-to-accurate depiction of the shade reading (shade analysis).

Step 5: fabricating the restoration (fabrication)

After assessing the shade, and determining what material works best given the particular clinical application (Fig. 18), the laboratory technician fabricates the restoration and adds the necessary details in the staining and glazing stage to match the opposing dentition (Fig. 19).

Step 6: verifying the accuracy of the shade match (verification)

Shade verification is one of the most critical phases of treatment. It should always be done in the laboratory by the laboratory technician before being returned to the clinician for try-in or insertion. The simplest means of shade verification is through the use of shade tabs. Using an 18% gray card as a background is also helpful to eliminate any surrounding distractions that could cause poor shade perception.

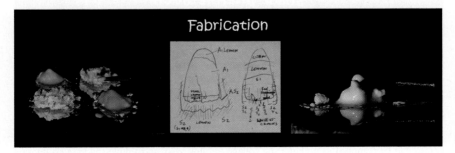

Fig. 18. The ceramist creates detailed tooth maps defining where the system's special effect powders should be used to achieve the desired nuances in shade.

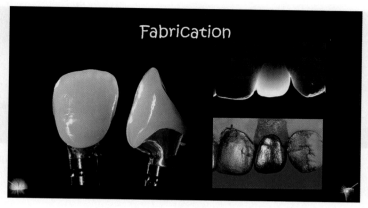

Fig. 19. Ceramic powders and internal colors are layered and stacked to proper shape, size, and contour to impart the correct visual effect on firing. Extrinsic glazes are added to finalize the color effects of the final restoration.

Step 7: placement (clinical insertion and cementation)

The ultimate verification of the restoration's accuracy happens when the clinician fits the restoration (Fig. 20). Does it or does it not match? If the restoration does not match, it should be a glaring problem. By using this protocol, however, remakes should be significantly minimized. If the restoration does not match, steps 2 through 6 should be repeated. The reference photographs should be taken with the new restoration in place and referenced accordingly.

Using the seven-step shade-taking and communication approach protocol, challenging anterior restorations can be matched confidently, predictably, and repeatedly (Fig. 21).

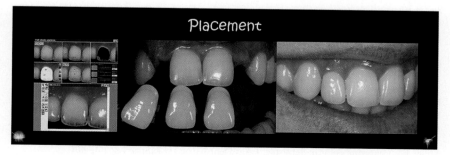

Fig. 20. Any discrepancies in the final restoration are immediately evident on placement by the clinician. Likewise, a perfect restoration appears indistinguishable among its natural neighbors.

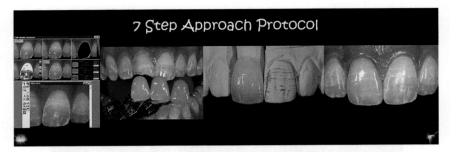

Fig. 21. Using the seven-step shade-taking and communication approach protocol, challenging anterior restorations can be matched confidently, predictably, and repeatedly.

Summary

The best way to analyze shade objectively is to use technology-based systems; however, shade tabs can be used judiciously. Details added by the laboratory technician in the fabrication process can often increase that natural appearance of a shade. This is best communicated with digital images and reference photography and an 18% gray card as the background to eliminate contrasting effects. Successful shade taking involves a combination of technology-based systems, shade tabs, and reference photography.

Further readings

A guide to understanding color communication. Grandville (MI): X-Rite; 2002.

Age-Related Eye Disease Study Research Group. A randomized placebo-controlled clinical trial of high-dose supplementation with vitamins C and E beta carotene and zinc for age-related macular degeneration and vision loss. AREDS report no. 8. Arch Ophthal 2001;119(10): 1417–36.

Carsten D. Successful shade matching: what does it take? Compend Contin Educ Dent 2003;24: 175–8, 180, 182.

Chu SJ, Devigus A, Mieleszko A. Fundamentals of color: shade matching and communication in esthetic dentistry. Chicago: Quintessence Publishing Co, Inc; 2004.

Chu SJ. Precision shade technology: contemporary strategies in shade selection. Pract Proced Aesthet Dent 2002;14:79–83.

Chu SJ. Science and art of porcelain veneers: color. Chicago: Quintessence Publishing; 2003. p. 157–206.

Chu SJ. The science of color and shade selection in aesthetic dentistry. Dent Today 2002;21(9): 86–9.

Commission Internationale de l'Eclairage. Colorimetry, official recommendations of the International Commission on Illumination. Publication CIE No. 15 (E-1.3.1). Paris: Bureau Central de la CIE; 1971.

Fraunfelder FT. Drug-induced ocular side effects. Philadelphia: Williams & Wilkins; 1996.

Hunter RS, Harold RW. The measurement of appearance. New York: Wiley; 1987. p. 3–68.

Kuehni RG, Marcus RT. An experiment in visual scaling of small color differences. Color Res Appl 1979;4:83–91.

Miller L. Organizing color in dentistry. J Am Dent Assoc 1987;[Spec Iss]:26E–40E.

Miller MD, Zaucha R. Color and tones. In: The color mac: design production techniques. Carmel (IN): Hayden; 1992. p. 23–39.

Munsell AH. A grammar of color. New York: Van Nostrand Dreinhold; 1969.

Paravina RD, Powers JM. Esthetic color training in dentistry. St. Louis (MO): Elsevier Mosby; 2004.

Rosenthal O, Phillips R. Coping with color-blindness. New York: Avery; 1997.

Sim CP, Yap AU, Teo J. Color perception among different dental personnel. Oper Dent 2001; 26(5):435–9.

Sproull RC. Color matching in dentistry, part I. The three-dimensional nature of color. J Prosthet Dent 1973;29:416–24.

Wasson W, Schuman N. Color vision and dentistry. Quintessence Int 1992;23(5):349–53.

Wyszecki G, Stiles WS. Color science concepts and methods, quantitative data and formulae. 2nd edition. New York: Wiley; 1982. p. 83–116.

THE DENTAL
CLINICS
OF NORTH AMERICA

Dent Clin N Am 51 (2007) 487–505

A Multidisciplinary Approach to Esthetic Dentistry

Frank M. Spear, DDS, MSD[a],
Vincent G. Kokich, DDS, MSD[b],*

[a]Seattle Institute for Advanced Dental Education, 600 Broadway, Seattle, WA 98122, USA
[b]Department of Orthodontics, University of Washington, Seattle, WA 98195, USA

In the past 25 years, the focus in dentistry has gradually changed. Years ago, dentists were in the repair business. Routine dental treatment involved excavating dental caries and filling of the enamel and dentinal defects with amalgam. In larger holes, more durable restorations may have been necessary, but the focus was the same: repair the effects of dental decay. However, with the advent of fluorides and sealants, in addition to the emergence of a better understanding of bacteria's role in causing both caries and periodontal disease, the needs of the dental patient have gradually changed. Many young adults who are products of the sealant generation have little or no decay and few existing restorations. At the same time, our image of the value of teeth in Western society has also changed. Yes, the public still regards teeth as an important part of chewing, but today the focus of many adults has shifted toward esthetics. How can my teeth be made to look better? Therefore, the formerly independent disciplines of orthodontics, periodontics, restorative dentistry, and maxillofacial surgery must often join together to satisfy the public's desire to look better.

This trend toward a heightened awareness of esthetics has challenged dentistry to look at dental esthetics in a more organized and systematic manner, so that the health of patients and their teeth is still the most important underlying objective. But some existing dentitions simply cannot be restored to a more pleasing appearance without the assistance of several different dental disciplines. Today, every dental practitioner must have a thorough understanding of the roles of these various disciplines in producing an esthetic makeover, with the most conservative and biologically sound interdisciplinary

* Corresponding author.
E-mail address: vgkokich@u.washington.edu (V.G. Kokich).

treatment plan possible. The authors have worked in such an environment for the past 20 years. As prosthodontist and orthodontist, we have belonged to an interdisciplinary study group consisting of nine dental specialists and one general dentist since 1984 [1]. We have met monthly since that time to (1) educate one another about the advances in each of our respective areas of dentistry and (2) to plan interdisciplinary treatment for some of the most challenging and complex dental situations. One of these interdisciplinary areas is esthetics. This article provides a systematic method of evaluating dentofacial esthetics in a logical, interdisciplinary manner.

Sequencing the planning process

Historically, the treatment planning process in dentistry usually began with an assessment of the biology or biological aspects of a patient's dental problem. This could include the patient's caries susceptibility, periodontal health, endodontic needs, and general oral health. Once the biologic health was reestablished either through caries removal, modification of the bone or gingiva, endodontic therapy, or tooth removal, then the restoration of the resulting defects would be based upon structural considerations. If teeth were to be restored or repositioned, the function of the teeth and condyles would be of paramount importance in dictating occlusal form and occlusal relationships, respectively. Finally, esthetics would be addressed to provide a pleasing appearance of the teeth. However, if the treatment planning sequence proceeds from biology to structure to function and finally to esthetics, the eventual esthetic outcome may be compromised. We proceed in the opposite direction. That is, we start the treatment planning process with esthetics and proceed to function, structure, and finally biology. We do not leave out any of the important parameters; we simply sequence the planning process from a different perspective. We choose this sequence because the decisions made in each category, especially esthetics, directly affect the following categories.

Beginning with esthetics in mind

When beginning with esthetics, we must begin with an appraisal of the position of the maxillary central incisors relative to the upper lip (Fig. 1). This assessment is made with the patient's upper lip at rest. Using a millimeter ruler or a periodontal probe, we determine the position of the incisal edge of the maxillary central incisor relative to the upper lip. The position of the maxillary central incisor can either be acceptable or unacceptable. An acceptable amount of incisal edge display at rest depends on the patient's age. Previous studies have shown that with advancing age, the amount of incisal display decreases proportionally [2,3]. For example, in a 30-year-old, 3 mm of incisal display at rest is appropriate. However, in a 60-year-old, the incisal display could be 1 mm or less. The change in incisal display

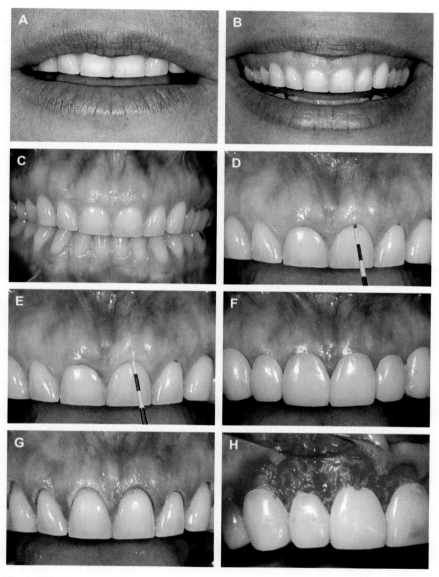

Fig. 1. This 35-year-old adult female showed about 3 mm of her maxillary central incisal edges with her lip at rest (*A*). However, she showed excessive gingiva when she smiled (*B*). Her occlusion was satisfactory, and she did not need orthodontic treatment (*C*). Her maxillary crown length was short, but the sulcus depth was normal (*D*). Sounding of the bone (*E*) showed that she had altered active eruption with the bone levels located at the cementoenamel junctions. A stent representing the desired crown length (*F*) was placed onto the upper teeth, and a gingivectomy was performed at that level (*G*). Then, a flap was elevated (*H*) showing the bone near the cementoenamel junction. The bone level was moved 3 mm above the desired gingival margins (*I*). After 5 years post-treatment (*J*), not only is the tissue healthy, but the ideal amount of gingiva is showing at rest (*K*) and during smiling (*L*).

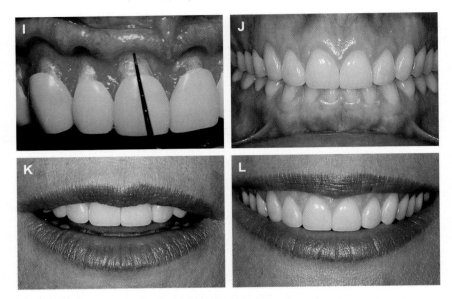

Fig. 1 (*continued*)

with time probably relates to the resiliency and tone of the upper lip, which tends to decrease with advancing age.

If the incisal edge display is inadequate (Fig. 2), then a primary objective of interdisciplinary treatment may be to lengthen the maxillary incisal edges. This objective could be accomplished with restorative dentistry [4], orthodontic extrusion [5], or orthognathic surgery [6–8]. Choosing the correct procedure depends upon the patient's facial proportions, existing crown length, and opposing occlusion. If the incisal edge display is excessive (Fig. 3), then an objective of treatment could be to move the maxillary incisors apically either by equilibration [9], restoration [10], orthodontics [11,12], or orthognathic surgery [13]. The selection among these disciplines again depends on the patient's existing anterior occlusion, the patient's facial proportions, or both.

The second aspect of esthetic tooth positioning to be evaluated is the maxillary dental midline. Recent studies have shown that lay people do not notice midline deviations to the right or left of up to 3 or 4 mm if the long axes of the teeth are parallel with the long axis of the face [14,15]. So, perhaps the most important relationship to evaluate is the medio-lateral inclination of the maxillary central incisors. If the incisors are inclined by 2 mm to the right or left, lay people regard this discrepancy as unesthetic [15,16]. A canted midline can be corrected with orthodontics [17] or restorative dentistry [18]. Usually the choice depends upon whether the maxillary incisors will require restoration.

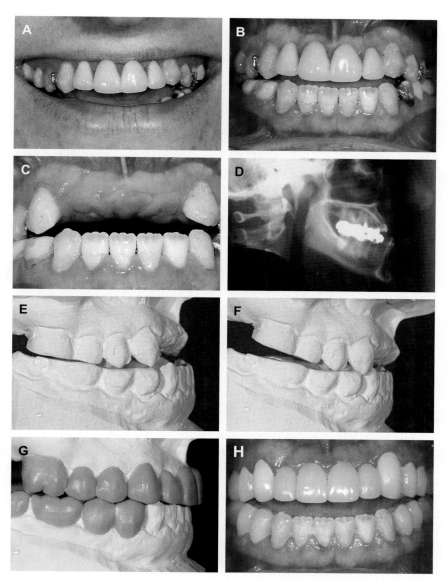

Fig. 2. This adult female lost her maxillary incisors in a childhood accident and was wearing a maxillary removable prosthesis (*A*). When smiling, her maxillary incisors were in the correct relationship relative to the upper lip, but the incisal edges were above the posterior occlusal plane (*B*), giving the patient an anterior openbite. Her past dental care was sporadic with decay and attrition noted in several areas (*C*). She had maxillary retrognathia (*D*). Orthognathic surgery was planned to move the maxillary posterior teeth apically to close the openbite but maintain the level of the maxillary incisal edges (*E* and *F*). A diagnostic wax-up (*G*) was used to fabricate provisional crowns, which were cemented (*H*) the day before jaw surgery. Orthodontic appliances were placed immediately before the surgery to stabilize the jaws after surgery (*I*). Implants were placed in the lateral incisor regions (*J*) and restored with a four-unit implant-supported bridge (*K*), which improved the patient's smile (*L*).

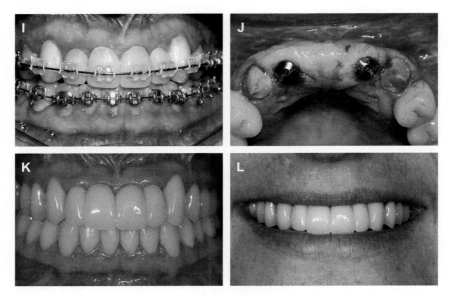

Fig. 2 (*continued*)

Maxillary incisor inclination

Once we have established the correct incisal edge position and midline relationship of the maxillary incisors, the next step is to evaluate the labiolingual inclination of the maxillary anterior teeth. Are they acceptable, proclined, or retroclined? When orthodontists evaluate labiolingual inclination, they rely on cephalometric radiographs to determine tooth inclination [19]. However, general dentists do not use these radiographs. Another method of assessing the inclination of the maxillary anterior teeth is to evaluate the labial surface of the existing maxillary central incisors relative to the patient's maxillary posterior occlusal plane. Generally, the labial surface of the maxillary central incisors should be perpendicular to the occlusal plane. This relationship permits maximum direct light reflection from the labial surface of the maxillary central incisors, which enhances their esthetic appearance [20]. If teeth are retroclined or proclined, correction may require either orthodontics or extensive restorative dentistry and possibly endodontics to establish a more ideal labiolingual inclination [18].

The next step is to evaluate the maxillary posterior occlusal plane relative to the ideal location of the maxillary incisal edge. Either the maxillary incisal edge will be level with the posterior occlusal plane (see Fig. 1; Figs. 4 and 5), coronal to the posterior occlusal plane (see Fig. 3; Fig. 6), or apical to the posterior occlusal plane (see Fig. 2). Correcting the posterior occlusal plane position requires orthognathic surgery [21,22], restorative dentistry [18], or both. The amount of tooth abrasion, the patient's vertical facial

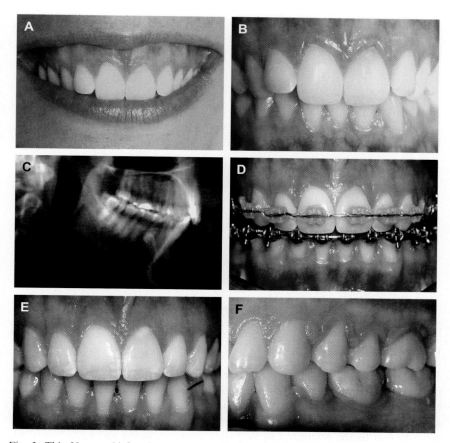

Fig. 3. This 30-year-old female was concerned about her "gummy smile" (*A*). She showed 5 mm of gingiva when she smiled, but the width-to-length relationship of her maxillary central incisors was ideal (*B*). She showed 8 mm of her maxillary incisors at rest (*C*) and, therefore, was diagnosed with maxillary alveolar hyperplasia. Orthodontics was used to coordinate the midlines (*D*), and maxillary impaction surgery was used to shorten her upper facial height and reduce the amount of gingiva. Her final occlusion (*E* and *F*) was improved significantly, and 5 years after orthodontic treatment, her smile still looks excellent (*G*) and her occlusion has been nicely maintained (*H* and *I*).

proportions, and the position of the alveolar bone help determine the correct solution for posterior occlusal plane discrepancies.

After the position of the maxillary central incisal edges have been determined, then the incisal edges of the maxillary lateral incisors and canines, as well as the buccal cusps of the maxillary premolars and molars can be established (see Fig. 2). The levels of these teeth generally are determined by their esthetic relationship to the lower lip when the patient smiles [23,24]. If the patient has an asymmetric lower lip, then it may be more prudent to use the interpupillary line as a guide in establishing the posterior occlusal plane [25].

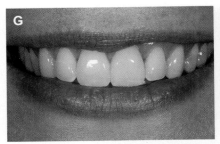
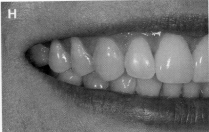

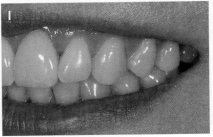

Fig. 3 (*continued*)

Determining the gingival levels

The next step in the process of determining the esthetic relationship of the maxillary anterior teeth is to establish the gingival levels. The current gingival levels should be assessed relative to the projected incisal edge position. The key to determining the correct gingival levels is to determine the desired tooth size relative to the projected incisal edge position (see Figs. 1, 2, 5, and 6). Remember that the incisal edge is not positioned to create the correct tooth size relative to the gingival margin levels. Using the gingiva as a reference to position the incisal edges is risky because gingiva can move with eruption or recession. So, the ideal gingival levels are determined by establishing the correct width-to-length ratio of the maxillary anterior teeth [26–28], by determining the desired amount of gingival display [15], and by establishing symmetry between right and left sides of the maxillary dental arch [18].

If the existing gingival levels will produce a tooth that is too short relative to the projected incisal edge position, then the gingival margins must be moved apically (see Figs. 1, 3, 5, and 6). This adjustment can either be accomplished with gingival or osseous surgery [29,30], through orthodontic intrusion [11], or with orthodontic intrusion and restoration [31–33]. The key factors that determine the most appropriate method of correction include the sulcus depth, the location of the cementoenamel junction relative to the bone level, the amount of existing tooth structure, the root-to-crown ratio, and the shape of the root [34]. In some situations, it is more appropriate to surgically crown-lengthen the maxillary incisors

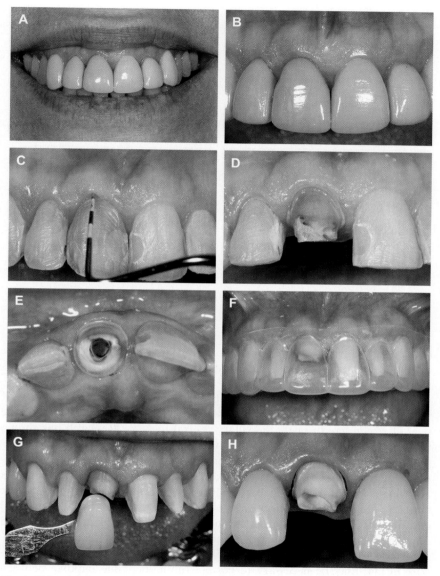

Fig. 4. This adult female was unhappy with the esthetics of her smile (*A*). The maxillary right central incisor had a nonvital pulp, and the root was dark (*B*). Her previous veneers were removed, and the tissue was probed over the maxillary right central incisor (*C*). After preparing the teeth, the right central incisor was very short (*D*), and the access opening for root-canal therapy was large (*E*), jeopardizing the structure of the teeth and the future restoration. The stent showed that preparation was adequate (*F*), and a shade guide was used to select the appropriate tooth color (*G*). The root fragment was bleached (*H*), and a post and coping was placed on the short tooth (*I*). The laboratory cast shows the extent of the restorations (*J*), and the size and shape of the crowns (*K*) and the esthetics of her smile (*L*) are improved.

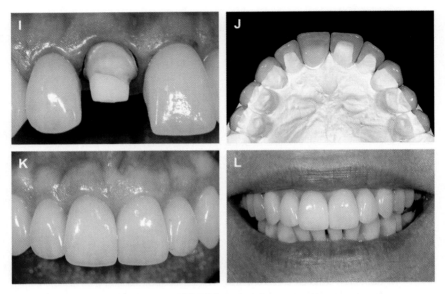

Fig. 4 (*continued*)

(see Fig. 1) to establish the correct gingival levels [10]. In other situations, orthodontic intrusion (see Fig. 5) and restoration of the incisal edge is more appropriate [34].

The next step in the process of establishing the correct esthetic position of the maxillary anterior teeth is to assess the papilla levels relative to the overall crown length of the maxillary central incisors. Research has shown that the average ratio is about 50% contact and 50% papilla [35]. If the contact is significantly shorter than the papilla (see Figs. 5 and 6), then moderate to significant incisor abrasion is likely, which tends to shorten the crowns and therefore shorten the contact between the central incisors [30]. If the contact is significantly longer than the papilla, then perhaps the gingival contour or scallop over the central incisors is flat (see Fig. 1), which could be caused by altered passive or altered active eruption of the teeth [36]. Either gingival or osseous surgery [10] or orthodontic intrusion [13] or extrusion [34] may be necessary to correct the level of the papillae between the maxillary anterior teeth.

Arrangement, contour, and shade

At this stage, the incisal edge position, the midline, the axial inclination, the gingival margins, and the papilla levels of the maxillary anterior teeth have been established. The next step is to determine if the arrangement of the maxillary anterior teeth can be accomplished restoratively. If not, will

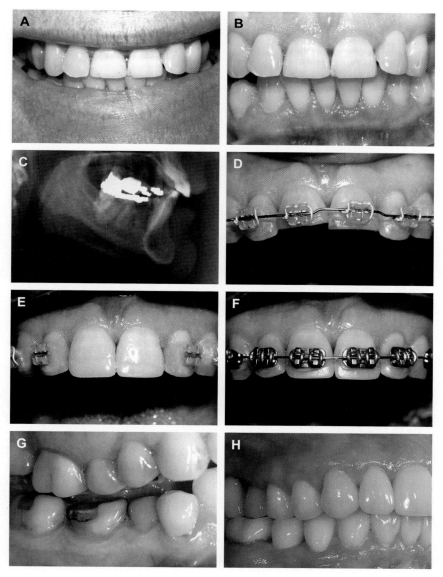

Fig. 5. (A–L) This adult female was unhappy with the appearance of her smile (A) and wanted longer maxillary anterior teeth (B). She had abraded her maxillary incisors, which had erupted to compensate and appeared short. The position of the maxillary incisal edge relative to the upper lip at rest was acceptable (C). Orthodontics was used to intrude the maxillary incisors (D) to move the gingival margins apically and provisionalize the teeth at a more attractive width-to-length proportion (E). Brackets were replaced on the maxillary incisors to stabilize them in their intruded position (F). Her posterior occlusion was improved during orthodontics (G and H) and her mandibular incisors were proclined labially to create coupling of the maxillary and mandibular anterior teeth during function. Space was opened to replace missing posterior teeth (J and K) and the esthetic appearance of her final restorations has been improved dramatically with interdisciplinary treatment (L).

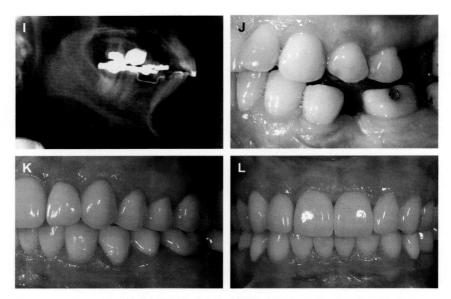

Fig. 5 (*continued*)

the patient require orthodontics to facilitate restoration? If in doubt, the clinician should perform a diagnostic wax-up (see Fig. 2) to confirm whether or not the arrangement is possible restoratively [18,34,37]. In addition, the contour and shade of the anterior teeth must be addressed. Does the patient have any specific requests concerning tooth shape or tooth shade? Remember, the more alterations made in these parameters, the more teeth will be treated, and the more involved the treatment plan will become. A good guide to esthetic treatment planning is to determine the ideal endpoint of treatment. Then compare it to the patient's current condition. Treatment is indicated when the desired endpoint and the current condition do not match. The actual method of treatment can then be chosen based upon the magnitude of the difference.

Develop the esthetic plan for the mandibular teeth

Now that the esthetic relationship of the maxillary incisors has been established, a proper relationship must be established between the mandibular incisors and the maxillary tooth position. First, evaluate the level of the mandibular incisal edges relative to the face. Do they have acceptable display, excessive display, or are they not visible? If they have excessive display, either equilibration, restoration, or orthodontic intrusion are possible methods of correcting the problem [34]. If they are not visible, either restoration or orthodontic extrusion may be necessary [38,39]. Next, determine

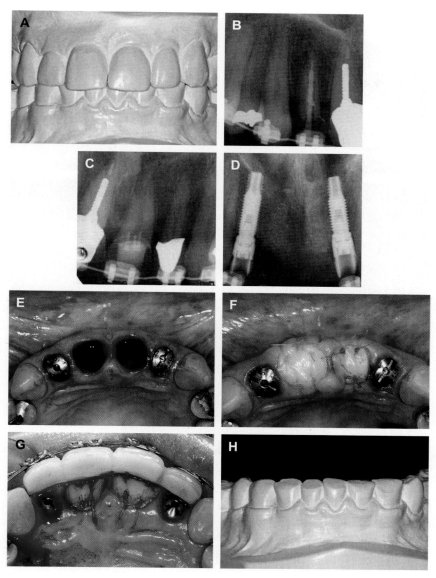

Fig. 6. This adult had short, worn, and hopeless maxillary incisors (*A*). Some of the teeth had failing root-canal therapy, and there was insufficient tooth structure remaining to restore these teeth (*B* and *C*). The maxillary central and lateral incisors were extracted and implants were placed in the lateral incisor positions (*D* and *E*). Tissue grafting was performed in the sockets of the extracted centrals to prepare the area for pontics (*F*). Since the orthodontic therapy was proceeding concurrently, a maxillary prosthesis was attached with brackets to the remaining teeth for esthetics (*G*). The mandibular incisors were abraded and had overerupted (*H*). These teeth were intruded nearly 3 mm (*I* and *J*) to avoid further reduction in height of these teeth during crown preparation. After the lower incisors were provisionalized with composite, brackets were replaced to stabilize tooth position (*K*). With adjunctive orthodontics, periodontics, implants, and coordinated therapy for this patient, the esthetics of her dentition and her occlusion were greatly improved (*L* and *M*).

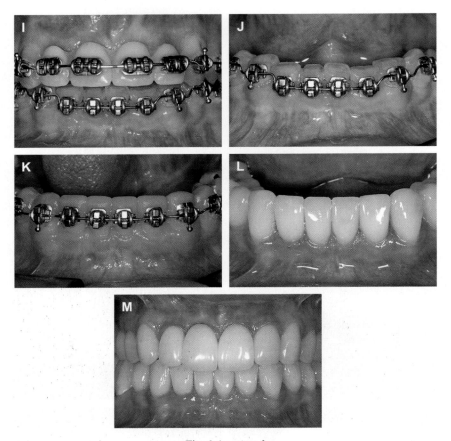

Fig. 6 (*continued*)

the relationship of the mandibular incisors relative to the posterior occlusal plane. Are the incisors level with the posterior occlusal plane? If not, then they are either coronal or apical to the posterior occlusal plane. Correcting either of these relationships could require restoration, equilibration, or orthodontics (see Fig. 6) [4]. Finally, the labiolingual inclination of the mandibular incisors must be evaluated. This relationship is partially determined by the projected position of the maxillary incisors. If the inclination is either proclined or retroclined (see Fig. 5), orthodontics could be a useful adjunct in adjusting the labiolingual position of the mandibular incisors [34]. The final mandibular incisal edge position is usually determined during the functional and structural phases of the treatment planning (see Figs. 5 and 6).

The gingival levels of the mandibular dentition may need to change when the different options for leveling the mandibular occlusal plane are considered. If orthodontics is selected to either intrude (see Fig. 6) or extrude teeth, the gingival margins move with the teeth [40]. However, if equilibration or restoration is necessary to level the mandibular occlusal plane, then the gingival levels may need to be relocated with osseous surgery [10].

At this point, based upon the esthetic determination of the projected positions of the maxillary and mandibular teeth, the clinician should be able to determine which teeth need restoration [41] (ie, the maxillary anteriors, maxillary posteriors, mandibular anteriors, or mandibular posteriors). Then, once the maxillary and mandibular occlusal planes have been established through esthetic parameters, the clinician must determine how to create an acceptable occlusal relationship between the arches.

Steps to integrating function and esthetics

The first step to integrating the esthetic plan with the functioning occlusion is to evaluate the temporomandibular joints and muscles [42]. Does the patient have any joint or muscle symptoms? A key step in the process is to make centric relation records and mount the models. Our definition of centric relation is the position of the condyles when the lateral pterygoid muscles are relaxed and the elevator muscles contact with the properly aligned disk [42]. The question that the clinician must ask is whether or not the desired esthetic changes can be made without altering the occlusion. If not, orthodontics or orthognathic surgery may be required to correct tooth position to facilitate the esthetic positioning of the teeth. To determine the impact of the esthetic plan on the function or occlusion, the esthetic changes in maxillary tooth position must be transferred to the maxillary dental cast [42]. This is accomplished with an application of wax in combination with an adjustment of the plaster casts (see Fig. 2).

As the proposed esthetic treatment plan is transferred to the mounted casts, the clinician can determine if restoration alone will accomplish the desired occlusion, or if alteration of the occlusal scheme through orthodontics or orthognathic surgery will be necessary. This is especially true when the clinician is planning to level the occlusal planes. A key question to ask is whether leveling of the occlusal planes creates an acceptable anterior dental relationship. If the answer is yes, and the leveling involves only the mandibular incisors, then the patient's existing vertical dimension can be maintained. If, however, the answer is no or the leveling involved mandibular posterior teeth, the existing vertical dimension may need to be altered. The clinician must determine whether altering the vertical dimension will result in acceptable tooth form and anterior relationships. There is no replacement for mounted dental casts and a diagnostic wax-up when these critical questions are being addressed.

Determine if adequate structure exists to restore teeth

Once the esthetic treatment plan has been established, the projected tooth position has been verified on the diagnostic wax-up, and the functional relationships of the mounted dental casts has been assessed, the clinician must determine if adequate tooth structure exists to restore the teeth. If not, how will the clinician obtain adequate structure? What types of restorations will be placed? How will they be retained? How will any missing teeth be replaced? Based upon the clinician's assessment of the remaining tooth structure [41], the choices for restoring anterior teeth could include composite bonding, porcelain veneers, bonded all-ceramic crowns, luted all-ceramic crowns, or metal ceramic crowns (see Figs. 1, 2, 4–6). The posterior restorations could include direct restorations, inlays, onlays, or crowns. If teeth are missing, they will either be replaced with implants, fixed partial dentures, or removable partial dentures. The evaluation criteria to determine which restorations are appropriate include (1) the current clinical crown length, (2) the crown length after any gingival changes are performed for esthetics, (3) current amount of ferrule [40], (4) the space available for a build-up, and (5) the effects on esthetics of any crown lengthening for structural purposes. The methods for increasing the retention of restorations are the build-up method, surgical crown lengthening [10], orthodontic forced eruption [33,40], and restorative bonding. Each clinical situation must be carefully evaluated to determine the appropriate structural solution.

Biology: last but certainly not least

The esthetic plan has been established. The diagnostic wax-up confirms that the teeth will function properly. The restorative plan has taken into consideration the existing tooth structure. Now is the time to add the biologic aspects of the treatment plan. The biologic aspects include endodontics, periodontics, and orthognathic surgery. The primary objective of biologic treatment planning is to establish a healthy oral environment with the tissue in the desired location. To accomplish this objective, endodontics may be necessary for teeth that are structurally and periodontally salvageable. In these cases, the endodontic therapy must be completed first, before beginning the restorative phase of dentistry. The definitive periodontal therapy must be established to create a healthy periodontium based upon the esthetic, functional, and structural needs of the restorations. Any elective periodontics must be completed next, in conjunction with the restorative plan. Finally, if there are any skeletal abnormalities that require orthognathic surgical correction, these must be accomplished before the definitive restorative phase of treatment.

Sequencing the therapy

The plan is complete. It began with esthetics, it was correlated to function, it took into consideration the remaining tooth structure, and it was facilitated by recognition of the biologic needs of the patient. The only two questions that remain are: (1) How should this esthetically based treatment plan be sequenced? and (2) Can the patient afford the treatment? The sequence of any treatment plan should always begin with the management or alleviation of acute problems. Then the remaining treatment plan can be sequenced in a manner that seems the most logical and facilitates the next or following phase of treatment, provided the result can be clearly identified, communicated, and achieved for the pertinent phase. When we establish the sequence of treatment for an interdisciplinary patient, we list the steps in the treatment plan based upon our collective opinion before the beginning of treatment [34,37]. Every member of the team receives a copy of the treatment sequence. This step ensures that each member of the team is able to follow the steps in the esthetic, functional, structural, and biologic rehabilitation of our mutual dental patient.

The economics of the interdisciplinary esthetic treatment plan is obviously of primary importance. To aid in this evaluation, it is useful to sort patients in four categories, as described in a previous article [43]. Type-I and -II patients generally do not require significant esthetic restoration. However, types III and IV typically require the type of esthetic evaluation that we have outlined in this article. The type-III patient is a healthy adult with no occlusal disease and no periodontal problems, but a desire for an esthetic change (see Figs. 1, 3, and 4). The type-III patient could be described as the cosmetic patient who is dentally healthy, but wishes to make a change in appearance. The hallmark of treating the true cosmetic patient is the requirement of time on the part of the dentist. The dentist must realize this commitment and charge a commensurate fee. The most challenging situation is the type-IV patient (see Figs. 2, 5, and 6), whom we have outlined in this article. This is an adult whose dentition is failing, may have occlusal disease, periodontal disease, multiple restorative needs, and missing teeth. The type-IV patient is the complex reconstruction patient in any dental practice. The hallmark of this patient is multiple appointments over months or even years, depending upon his or her orthodontic, periodontal, endodontic, surgical, and restorative needs. Due to the increased number of appointments and lab fees, the clinician must adjust the fees to reflect the amount of time commitment. For ideas on establishing appropriate fees in these types of patients, the reader is referred to this previous article [43].

Summary

Esthetics has become a respectable term in dentistry. In the past, the importance of esthetics was discounted in favor of terms such as function, structure, and biology. However, if a treatment plan does not begin with a clear view of its esthetic impact on the patient, then the outcome could be disastrous. In today's interdisciplinary dental world, treatment planning must begin with well-defined esthetic objectives. By beginning with esthetics, and taking into consideration the impact on function, structure, and biology, the clinician can use the various disciplines in dentistry to deliver the highest level of dental care to each patient. It really works. We call this process interdisciplinary esthetic dentistry.

References

[1] Spear F. My growing involvement in dental study groups. J Am Coll Dent 2002;69:22–4.
[2] Vig RG, Brundo GC. The kinetics of anterior tooth display. J Prosthet Dent 1978;39:502–4.
[3] Ackerman MB, Brensinger C, Landis JR. An evaluation of dynamic lip-tooth characteristics during speech and smile in adolescents. Angle Orthod 2004;74:43–50.
[4] Spear F, Kokich VG, Mathews D. An interdisciplinary case report. Advanced Esthetics and Interdisciplinary Dentistry 2005;1(2):12–8.
[5] Lopez-Gavito G, Wallen TR, Little RM, et al. Openbite malocclusion: a longitudinal 10-year post-retention evaluation of orthodontically treated patients. Am J Orthod 1985; 87:175–86.
[6] De Mol van Otterloo JJ, Tuinzing DB, Kostense P. Inferior positioning of the maxilla by a Le Fort I osteotomy: a review of 25 patients with vertical maxillary deficiency. J Craniomaxillofac Surg 1996;24:69–77.
[7] Major PW, Phillippson GE, Glover KE, et al. Stability of maxilla downgrafting after rigid or wire fixation. J Oral Maxillofac Surg 1996;54:1287–91.
[8] Costa F, Robiony M, Zerman N, et al. Bone biological plate for stabilization of maxillary inferior repositioning. Minerva Stomatol 2005;54:227–36.
[9] Kokich VG. Maxillary lateral incisor implants: planning with the aid of orthodontics. J Oral Maxillofac Surg 2004;62:48–56.
[10] Spear F. Construction and use of a surgical guide for anterior periodontal surgery. Contemporary Esthetics and Restorative Practice 1999;12–20.
[11] Kokich VG. Anterior dental esthetics. An orthodontic perspective II. Vertical relationships. J Esthet Dent 1993;5:174–8.
[12] Nanda R. Correction of deep overbite in adults. Dent Clin North Am 1997;41:67–87.
[13] Kokich VG, Spear FM, Kokich VO. Maximizing anterior esthetics: an interdisciplinary approach. In: McNamara JA Jr, editor. Frontiers in dental and facial esthetics. Ann Arbor (MI): Craniofacial Growth Series, Center for Human Growth and Development, Needham Press, University of Michigan; 2001. p. 2–19.
[14] Beyer JW, Lindauer SJ. Evaluation of dental midline position. Semin Orthod 1998;4: 146–52.
[15] Kokich VO, Kiyak HA, Shapiro PA. Comparing the perception of dentists and lay people to altered dental esthetics. J Esthet Dent 1999;11:311–24.
[16] Thomas JL, Hayes C, Zawaideh S. The effect of axial midline angulation on dental esthetics. Angle Orthod 2003;73:359–64.
[17] Kokich VG. Anterior dental esthetics: an orthodontic perspective III. Mediolateral relationships. J Esthet Dent 1993;5:200–7.
[18] Spear FM. The esthetic correction of anterior dental mal-alignment: conventional vs. instant (restorative) orthodontics. J Calif Dent Assoc 2004;32:133–41.
[19] Littlefield K. A review of the literature of selected cephalometric analyses. St. Louis (MO): St. Louis University Press; 1992.
[20] Rufenacht C. Fundamentals of esthetics. Carol Stream (IL): Quintessence Publishing; 1990.
[21] Denison TF, Kokich VG, Shapiro PA. Stability of maxillary surgery in openbite versus nonopenbite malocclusions. Angle Orthod 1989;59:5–10.
[22] Proffit WR, Bailey LJ, Phillips C, et al. Long-term stability of surgical open-bite correction by Le Fort I osteotomy. Angle Orthod 2000;70:112–7.
[23] Naylor CK. Esthetic treatment planning: the grid analysis system. J Esthet Restor Dent 2002;14:76–84.

[24] van der Geld PA, van Waas MA. The smile line: a literature search. Ned Tijdschr Tand-heelkd 2003;110:350–4.

[25] Chiche G, Kokich V, Caudill R. Diagnosis and treatment planning of esthetic problems. In: Pinault A, Chiche G, editors. Esthetics in fixed prosthodontics. Carol Stream (IL): Quintes-sence; 1994. p. 33–52.

[26] Gillen RJ, Schwartz RS, Hilton TJ, et al. An analysis of selected normative tooth propor-tions. Int J Prosthodont 1994;7:410–7.

[27] Sterrett JD, Oliver T, Robinson F, et al. Width/length ratios of normal clinical crowns of the maxillary anterior dentition in man. J Clin Periodontol 1999;26:153–7.

[28] Wolfart S, Thormann H, Freitag S, et al. Assessment of dental appearance following changes in incisor proportions. Eur J Oral Sci 2005;113:159–65.

[29] Kokich VG. Esthetics: the ortho-perio-restorative connection. Seminars in Orthodontics and Dentofacial Orthopedics 1996;2:21–30.

[30] Kokich VG, Kokich VO. Orthodontic therapy for the periodontal-restorative patient. In: Rose L, Mealey B, Genco R, et al, editors. Periodontics: medicine, surgery, and implants. St. Louis (MO): Mosby-Elsevier; 2004. p. 718–44.

[31] Kokich VG. Anterior dental esthetics: an orthodontic perspective I. Crown length. J Esthet Dent 1993;5:19–23.

[32] Kokich VG. Esthetics and vertical tooth position: the orthodontic possibilities. Compend Contin Educ Dent 1997;18:1225–31.

[33] Kokich VG. Managing orthodontic—restorative treatment for the adolescent patient. In: McNamara JA Jr, editor. Orthodontics and dentofacial orthopedics. Ann Arbor (MI): Needham Press, Inc.; 2001. p. 395–422.

[34] Kokich VG, Kokich VO. Interrelationship of orthodontics with periodontics and restorative dentistry. In: Nanda R, editor. Biomechanics and esthetic strategies in clinical orthodontics. St. Louis (MO): Elsevier Press; 2005. p. 348–73.

[35] Kurth J, Kokich VG. Open gingival embrasures after orthodontic treatment in adults: prevalence and etiology. Am J Orthod Dentofacial Orthop 2001;120:116–23.

[36] Spear F. Maintenance of the interdental papilla following anterior tooth removal. Pract Periodontics Aesthet Dent 1999;11:21–8.

[37] Kokich VG, Spear F. Guidelines for treating the orthodontic-restorative patient. Seminars in Orthodontics and Dentofacial Orthopedics 1999;3:3–20.

[38] Emerich-Poplatek K, Sawicki L, Bodal M, et al. Forced eruption after crown/root fracture with a simple and aesthetic method using the fractured crown. Dent Traumatol 2005;21: 165–9.

[39] Koyuturk AE, Malkoc S. Orthodontic extrusion of subgingivally fractured incisor before restoration. A case report: 3-years follow-up. Dent Traumatol 2005;21:174–8.

[40] Spear F. When to restore and when to remove the tooth. Insight and Innovation 2001;29–37.

[41] Spear F. A conversation with Dr. Frank Spear. Dental Practitioner Report 2002;42–8.

[42] Spear F. Occlusion in the new millennium: the controversy continues. Signature 2002;7: 18–21.

[43] Spear F. Implementing the plan: the economics of restorative dentistry. Insight and Innova-tion 2001;33–40.

ELSEVIER
SAUNDERS

Dent Clin N Am 51 (2007) 507–524

THE DENTAL
CLINICS
OF NORTH AMERICA

Esthetic Considerations when Splinting with Fiber-Reinforced Composites

Howard E. Strassler, DMD[a],*, Cheryl L. Serio, DDS[b]

[a]*Department of Endodontics, Prosthodontics and Operative Dentistry, University of Maryland Dental School, 650 West Baltimore Street, Baltimore, MD 21201, USA*
[b]*Department of Care Planning and Restorative Sciences, University of Mississippi School of Dentistry, 2500 North State Street, Jackson, MS 39216-4505, USA*

Fiber-reinforced composite resins are highly filled composite resins that are strengthened with the use of embedded fiber threads [1]. There are a number of fiber reinforcement materials available for providing dental resin reinforcement in clinical situations (Table 1). Fiber-reinforcement materials can be made from polyethylene yarns woven to create a ribbon, glass fibers woven to create a ribbon, and short and long strands of glass fibers embedded in a resin matrix (preimpregnated glass fibers). In all cases, there are surface treatments of the fibers that allow them to bond to dental resins [1,2]. Glass fibers are pretreated with organo-silanes that act as chemical coupling agents between dental resin and the glass. Woven fiber ribbons made from high-molecular-weight, high-tensile strength, biocompatible, color-neutral polyethylene are plasma treated. The plasma treatment of the fibers ablates (etches) and chemically activates the fibers to allow them to chemically bond to dental resins, creating a polymeric hybrid that functions as a laminate. The glass and polyethylene fiber reinforcement of the dental resin–fiber network exhibit the characteristics necessary for a load-bearing area even in a thin veneer. In a recent Consensus Conference on fiber reinforcement materials, it was demonstrated that fiber reinforcement materials for composite resins are a highly successful restorative treatment modality and enhance dental care [3].

Fiber reinforcement within composite resins have a variety of uses that include splinting of teeth [4], restoration of the endodontically treated tooth [5], and cross splinting teeth that contain large composite restorations [6].

Portions of this article were adapted from Strassler HE, Garber DA. Anterior esthetic considerations when splinting teeth. Dent Clin North Am 43(1):167–78, 1999.
    * Corresponding author.
    E-mail address: hstrassler@umaryland.edu (H.E. Strassler).

doi:10.1016/j.cden.2006.12.004

Table 1
Partial listing fiber reinforcement materials for directly placed composite resin splints

Product (manufacturer)	Type of fiber (widths)
everStickC&B, everStickPerio everStick Ortho (Stick Tech, Turku, Finland)	2 cm preimpregnated glass bundle
everStickNet (Stick Tech)	1×30-cm^2 preimpregnated glass fabric sheet
Ribbond Reinforcement Ribbon (Ribbond, Seattle, WA)	Lock-stitch, woven polyethylene (1 mm, 2 mm, 3 mm, 4 mm, and 9 mm)
Ribbond THM ribbon (Ribbond)	Lock-stitch, woven polyethylene (1 mm ortho, 2 mm, 3 mm, 4 mm, and 7 mm)
Ribbond Triaxial (Ribbond)	Three axis braided weave, polyethylene fiber ribbon (dense, thin)
Connect (Kerr, Orange, CA)	Open-weave, polyethylene ribbon (2 mm and 3 mm)
Splint-It (Pentron, Wallingford, CT)	Open-weave, glass fiber ribbon (2 mm); unidirectional, glass fiber ribbon (3 mm)
DVA (Dental Ventures of America, Riverside, CA)	Open tufts of polyethylene fibers
GlasSpan rope (GlasSpan, Exton, PA)	Open-weave glass fiber ribbon and (4 mm ribbon, 2 mm, and 3 mm rope)

The most common use for fiber reinforcement that has been described in the dental literature has been the splinting of teeth [4,7,8]. A splint, as defined by the *Glossary of Prosthodontic Terms*, is "a device that maintains hard and/or soft tissue in a predetermined position" [9]. Teeth are splinted for a variety of reasons, including to replace missing teeth, to retain teeth that have been orthodontically repositioned, to stabilize teeth that have been traumatized, and to stabilize teeth that are periodontally involved and have mobility.

When teeth are joined together for the purpose of splinting, stabilization, or restoration as a result of missing teeth, the technical elements of marginal fit, correct contour and shape of the restoration, cleansibility, and occlusion must be fulfilled. In the esthetic zone of the oral cavity, an acceptable cosmetic result must be achieved. Clinically, a splint can be a cast-fixed or removable partial denture or a reinforced adhesive composite resin restoration. A splint joins teeth together with the treatment goal of stabilization, and the connection between the teeth must be strong enough to withstand the forces of mastication and the parafunctional forces of grinding, clenching, and trauma. When anterior teeth are splinted, thorough treatment planning is essential to fulfill the need for a long-term durable restoration without compromising esthetic goals. Therefore, the clinician must design the tooth preparations and subsequent restorations, taking into account the connector areas, interproximal contact areas, incisal/occlusal embrasures, and gingival spaces.

The primary focus of dental care is the treatment of pathologic conditions of the oral hard and soft tissues. The goal of treatment is to establish a physiologically stable result that can be maintained in a healthy state by the patient. At times, treatment results may compromise patient esthetics. How important is the final esthetic result? Lombardi [10] stated that dental esthetics is the most important aspect of all of the dental specialties, including pediatric dentistry, orthodontics, oral surgery, periodontics, and restorative dentistry. He further described physical attractiveness as playing an essential role in one's self-esteem and as being an important concept for the entire dental team [10]. Dentists have the ability to increase the attractiveness of a patient's smile, which may change a patient's life as self-confidence improves. The physiologic implications of esthetic dental treatment to preserve or restore a person's self-image, self-esteem, and well-being have been well documented [11]. Patients sometimes neglect their oral health until dental disease has a direct impact on their physical appearance. Although a patient's goal may be to restore the esthetic function of the teeth, this should not compromise overall dental health [12]. It is the dentist's ultimate responsibility to preserve, enhance, or create a pleasing smile through dental treatment but not at the expense of function. Sometimes the patient's goal is elimination of dental pain; however, the dentist must not fail to discuss the esthetic implications of a proposed plan of treatment [13]. It is the responsibility of the practitioner to provide a comprehensive treatment plan to the patient, discuss the treatment goals, and strive to attain all treatment goals.

Evaluation of the esthetic zone

The goal patients is that there be a normal esthetic relationship linking the appearance of the teeth, gingival tissues and supporting structures, and the oromaxillofacial complex. From a physiologic standpoint, a smile can be portrayed as a change in the oral musculature that raises the lips at the corners of the mouth into a curve that generally exposes some of the teeth. The amount of tooth structure that can be visualized is dependent on the retraction of the lips from the teeth. In some cases, people expose minimal gingival tissues; however, in other cases, a broad smile reveals all of the gingival tissues. In most cases, when teeth are not splinted together, each tooth has an individualized appearance. Once teeth are joined together through splinting, the connectors change the three-dimensional appearance of the interproximal spaces and the individuality of each tooth.

The esthetic appearance of teeth is a mixture of each individual tooth shape, the position of the teeth within the dental arch, and the interrelationships of the teeth to the opposing dental arch. Depending on tooth position, teeth can create an agreeable or disagreeable visual appearance. The psychologic responses to a person's smile by others is a blend of complex visual judgments. Within each culture, there are norms regarding what constitutes a pleasing smile. For those who believe their smile is unattractive due to disharmonious tooth position, color, shape, or contours, the oral musculature has been trained to cover the teeth when the person smiles. Even though the

lips and corners of the mouth are turning in an upward direction, the teeth
are guarded and therefore hidden from view by the oral musculature.

A smile is a combination of the appearance of each tooth, the appearance
of the teeth and adjacent gingival tissues as a unit, and how all of these are
framed by the oral musculature and lips. In the anterior zone, the maxillary
incisors are usually the teeth seen when one smiles. These teeth can have
a variety of shapes and forms. Theories of tooth forms and facial profiles
led to the description and selection of teeth based upon different tooth forms
[14]. From these theories, denture tooth manufacturers classified tooth
forms based upon specific descriptions of maxillary incisor shapes. These descriptions include tapering, ovoid, square, square ovoid, and square tapering. Research has shown that there is no correlation between tooth form
and facial profile, but these descriptions persist [14]. The basic shape of
a tooth is also affected by the facial surface contours, the length and width
of the tooth, the position of the facial line angles of the tooth, and the surface texture of the tooth and how it reflects light. Tooth color (shade) is an
important facet of the esthetic appearance, especially in this era of tooth
whitening. Shades approaching white that were once considered too high
in value are now considered normal.

Not only are individual tooth form and color important in the esthetic
appearance; how the teeth appear as a group is also important. Within
a dental arch, the teeth in the esthetic zone are visualized through the
appearance of tooth individualization, tooth arrangement, appearance of
each tooth relative to its companion teeth [14], and the appearance of the
gingival tissues [15]. These critical factors include gingival color and contour, midline, tooth size proportion, tooth position, incisal lengths, tooth
widths, axial inclination, occlusal plane, and interproximal relationships
between teeth.

Healthy gingival tissues have a pleasing appearance and frame the teeth
to which they are attached. Gingival tissues that are inflamed and hyperplastic are detractors to a pleasing smile. Healthy gingival tissue adapts to the
necks of the teeth and follows the contours of the cementoenamel junction
of the teeth and the underlying bone. There is considerable variation in the
appearance of gingival tissues relative to tooth position, gingival pigmentation, and thickness of the gingival tissues [15]. In the case of a missing tooth,
the gingival shape of the ridge can have a variety of forms due to the reason
for tooth loss, the type of surgical procedure required for extraction, or the
absence of tooth formation in the ridge area.

Tooth-to-tooth relationships have a direct impact on esthetic appearance.
The arrangement of anterior and adjacent teeth in the esthetic zone is the
most dominant factor influencing esthetics [16]. In most cases, teeth and
smiles are viewed at right angles to the facial surfaces of the maxillary incisors. When one views one's own teeth, it is generally in a mirror at right
angles. The cosmetic appearance of a smile is directly influenced by a society's
expectations for an attractive smile. The most appealing features of a smile

as it is framed by the lips and the face are symmetry and proportion [17]. Most people do not have "perfect" symmetry and proportion.

Within the limitations of dental treatment, there are goals that can be accomplished when providing esthetic tooth splinting. An esthetically pleasing appearance can be achieved by having the midline coincide with other centered features of the face (ie, the nose, philtrum, and chin). When splinting teeth, the design of the interproximal connector should be based upon tooth width and length to create a proportional appearance. Splinted teeth are more esthetically pleasing when the incisal edges are aligned without tooth rotations, overlap, or facial or lingual positioning with respect to the arch form. When teeth are splinted, it is important to individualize the appearance of the teeth by creating incisal embrasure spaces without oversilhouetting the light appearance of the teeth against the darker areas of the intraoral cavity [16].

When viewing the maxillary anterior teeth, the relationship of the occlusal plane to the incisal line of the teeth plays an important role in defining an esthetically pleasing smile. Typically, this is defined by the relationship of the incisal line of the maxillary anterior teeth extending to the facial cusp tips of the posterior teeth. In most cases, the incisal line of the maxillary central incisors should be parallel to the interpupillary line, with the maxillary lateral incisal edges slightly more apical in position, denoting a positive smile line [18].

In some cases, these "rules" cannot be followed due to the limitations of tooth position, arch space and size, tooth shape and size, and occlusion. During a treatment plan, these limitations need to be explained to the patient. The choice of treatment by the patient may be dictated by their expectation of a desired final result. Major tooth shape, size, color, and alignment issues may be treated best with conventional fixed partial dentures and not fiber-reinforced composites.

Esthetics and splinted teeth

The challenge in creating or maintaining an esthetically pleasing restorative result when splinting teeth is to duplicate those factors that provide an esthetic result when teeth are not joined together. A fixed partial denture is usually the treatment of choice to replace a missing tooth. Frequently, periodontally involved teeth are splinted to control increasing tooth mobility associated with secondary occlusal trauma.

When teeth are joined together with a connector, the result usually produces an artificial esthetic barrier to the three-dimensional appearance of teeth. For a splint to be successful and durable, the connectors between the splinted teeth must have a specific thickness of restorative material to resist fracture in normal function and parafunction. Connectors used for splinting teeth include cast metal, cast metal covered with ceramic, composite resin with embedded fiber ribbon, metal bars or wires, and nylon mesh.

Teeth with spacing present an additional esthetic dilemma. If the spaces are to be maintained, the connector used for splinting must be placed so it is not visually apparent.

In most cases, the optimal placement of the interproximal connector from a facial view when splinting is on the incisal/occlusal or middle third of the tooth. This location mimics the presence of the interproximal contact area between adjacent teeth. This location also provides access for the clinician to shape the restoration and reestablish an esthetic result. The management of the incisal/occlusal embrasures, facial interproximal connector areas, and the gingival embrasures is important to achieve desirable esthetics and function. When planning a splint or fixed partial denture, the lingual surfaces of the restored teeth must be designed to have adequate thickness for the bulk of the restorative material to resist the forces of occlusion and mastication. In some cases, it may be necessary to reshape opposing teeth to establish occlusal patterns that allow the connector to have the required thickness for clinical durability.

The placement of the connector in the incisal/occlusal or middle third of the tooth is important in the establishment of an esthetic and hygienic gingival embrasure [19]. The gingival embrasure must be designed so that the patient has access to remove plaque to maintain periodontal health and prevent caries.

The type of splint being planned has a major impact on the final esthetic appearance of the case. In clinical situations where a porcelain–metal or all ceramic restoration is planned, tooth preparations allow for easier and better esthetic and occlusal control of the final result. The esthetic limitations of splinted teeth are minimized with a laboratory-fabricated, fixed partial denture. When a fiber–reinforced, direct composite resin is being placed, the conservation of tooth structure for a predictable bonding surface of enamel [20] requires more complex treatment planning by the clinician to achieve an esthetic final result. It is critical that the clinician observe the esthetic needs of the case in the planning and tooth modification required from several important esthetic dimensions: incisal embrasure form, facial and interproximal embrasure form, and gingival embrasure form. These aspects in planning and restoration are demonstrated through several cases of splinting using fiber reinforcement.

Incisal embrasure form

The incisal embrasures are critical for the esthetic silhouette of the incisal edges of maxillary and mandibular teeth. If each tooth is not individualized by carving this feature into the splint, the teeth have a block-like appearance. This loss of individuality decreases the illusion of spacing. Using tooth contour with the establishment of definitive incisal embrasures improves the facial appearance of the teeth in profile. Designing incisal embrasures outlines the difference in heights and separation of the maxillary incisal edges and differentiates each mandibular incisor as a separate entity. Otherwise, the teeth appear as one solid block without distinction between each tooth. In the maxillary arch, the incisal embrasure between the central incisors is in most cases approximately 1.0 mm lower than the embrasures between the central and lateral incisors. The incisal embrasure between the lateral incisor and canine is generally longer because of the change in shape between the more square or tapered lateral incisor and the more triangular incisal appearance of the canine. The embrasure form of the mandibular incisors, although not as prominent as the maxillary incisors, is just as important in creating a natural visual impact through incisal separation [21]. As we get older and the incisal edges wear, the incisal embrasure decreases and eventually can vanish, leaving the block-like appearance [14].

With these factors in mind, the design of the restoration has to allow for adequate incisal embrasure without compromising strength and durability in the connector of the restoration. For cast porcelain–metal and all-ceramic restorations, the tooth preparation must allow for the design of the framework so that final porcelain application can be accomplished, allowing each tooth to be distinct from the adjacent teeth. The final crown preparation must take this into account so that the framework in the incisal area of the connector allows for at least 1.0 to 1.2 mm of porcelain covering the metal or ceramic substructure. For reinforced, bonded composite resin splints, the reinforcement ribbon must be placed so that at least 1.0 mm of composite resin remains after esthetic carving of the incisal embrasure form. Less thickness of the composite resin can lead to premature fracture and exposure of the fibers. Shaping should be accomplished, creating incisal embrasure form from the lingual and facial surfaces so that the final tooth form from an incisal view is maintained.

Facial and interproximal form

The three-dimensional illusion of the teeth within a splinted restoration is achieved by careful design of the tooth preparations. In the case of porcelain–metal or all-ceramic restorations, the tooth reduction creates the room for the overlying metal or ceramic substructure with the esthetic porcelain applied. Typical crown preparations easily allow for these requirements for the final restoration. For conservative fiber-reinforced splinted restorations, there are limitations to the amount of tooth structure that can be prepared based upon the tooth substrate to be bonded to (preferably enamel) and the existing occlusion. Evaluation of occlusion to fulfill the requirements of the fiber-reinforced composite must be done in maximum intercuspation and in excursive movements. If interferences are created when the definitive restoration is fabricated, the teeth must be modified by preparation to eliminate the potential for these interferences. This must be done as part of the diagnosis and treatment planning phase using casts mounted on an articulator.

After a comprehensive evaluation, decisions must be made on how the tooth shapes need to be modified and prepared to allow for an esthetic interproximal and facial embrasure form that does not compromise the durability of the definite fiber-reinforced splint. In contrast to porcelain–metal and all-ceramic fixed partial denture splints, composite resin restorations are more susceptible to fatigue failure. By using reinforcement materials embedded within the composite, such as woven polyethylene ribbon or unidirectional glass fibers, the potential fracture and separation of the splint can be overcome [22]. When reinforcement ribbon and composite resin is used for splinting, the physical properties of the laminated structure can be maximized by placing the ribbon in the tensile zone of the splint [1].

For maxillary periodontal splints, definitive tooth preparation of the facial surface to compensate for thickness of fiber ribbon reinforcement and composite is necessary to eliminate the overcontouring of the final restoration. Facial placement of the fiber also allows for maintaining occlusion on tooth rather than composite [23,24]. In the case of a periodontal splint, there is concern that the patient will wear the lingual surface of the composite resin into the fiber reinforcement, leaving the fibers exposed and compromising the durability of the splint. For cases of direct single-tooth replacement with a fiber-reinforced, composite, fixed partial denture for the maxillary arch, the use of Class 3 preparations on the adjacent abutment teeth and a lingual channel with adequate depth to place the fiber closer to the facial surface and the tensile zone is necessary.

To achieve facial and interproximal individualization of teeth, it is necessary that tooth preparation for maxillary and mandibular fiber splints barrel into one half of the interproximal contact area using a medium-grit diamond on the high-speed handpiece. This facial preparation minimizes bulk on the esthetic facial surface interproximally and allows the composite resin to have adequate thickness for strength while allowing it to be shaped for esthetic individualization of each tooth that is splinted. Other purposes for the placement of facial composite resin are to seal the interproximal areas against recurrent caries, to provide for a 180° wrap of composite resin to each of the splinted teeth, and to stabilize the teeth to prevent movement when the composite resin and ribbon are placed onto the lingual surface for mandibular splints. For maxillary periodontal splints, some additional interproximal preparation is necessary so that the fiber reinforcement material can be pushed and embedded within the interproximal contact area, allowing for room to shape an esthetic composite resin in the connector area. This facial extension of composite resin also functions as a cross-splint for each tooth to prevent tooth movement and breakage of the final splint.

When the fiber-reinforced composite resin is light cured, shaping and individualization of each tooth in the connector area can be accomplished with ultrathin, needle-shaped diamonds with a high-speed handpiece; with thin disks with a slow-speed handpiece; or with a reciprocating handpiece (Profin; Dentatus, New York, NY) with thin, flat, safe-sided, diamond-

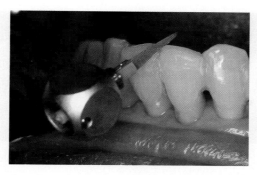

Fig. 1. Using the Profin reciprocating handpiece with a flat, safe-sided diamond abrasive Lamineer "S" tip to shape the incisal embrasure of a Ribbond fiber–reinforced periodontal splint. (*Adapted from* Strassler HE, Garber DA. Anterior esthetic considerations when splinting teeth. Dent Clin North Am 1999;43(1):167–78; with permission.).

impregnated Lamineer tips (Fig. 1). The experience of these authors is that the reciprocating handpiece is less problematic in forming these facial embrasure areas because of its precision for fine shaping in these areas.

Gingival form

Just as important as tooth form and individuality of the facial interproximal areas at the connectors and the incisal embrasure form is the gingival embrasure. When designing a splinted restoration, the gingival embrasure form must allow for maintenance of gingival health. The pink-stippled gingival appearance contributes to the overall esthetic appearance of the restoration. If the patient cannot maintain the gingiva with oral hygiene procedures, the gingiva can develop an erythematous, edematous appearance that detracts from the esthetic appearance of the final restoration.

In the case of the replacement of a long-standing missing tooth in the esthetic zone, the pontic shape should have a light contact on the ridge. Recontouring the gingival ridge to create an ovate pontic emerging from the

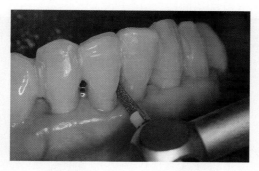

Fig. 2. Using the Profin reciprocating handpiece with a flat, safe-sided diamond abrasive Lamineer "S" tip to shape the gingival embrasure of a Ribbond fiber–reinforced periodontal splint.

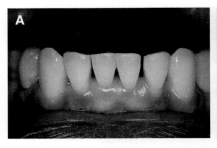
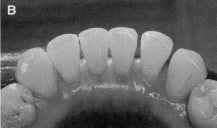

Fig. 3. Preoperative view of mandibular anterior teeth with Grade 2 mobility. (*A*) Facial view. (*B*) Lingual view.

ridge is recommended [25]. This emergence profile of the pontic should mimic the contours of the adjacent teeth. Another significant gingival esthetic problem is the presence of a localized defect on the ridge. Before fabrication of the definitive fixed partial denture to replace the missing tooth or teeth, a surgical technique similar to that used in root coverage procedures using a soft connective tissue graft to eliminate the defect has been successful [26]. Also, the facial form of the pontic must match the analogous tooth in the arch in shape and size and disguise the interdental space. The physical requirements of the connector must also be taken into account.

In many cases, the use of a direct-placement, fiber-reinforced, fixed partial denture is recommended for sudden tooth loss in the esthetic zone of the anterior region usually due to trauma, periodontal disease, or endodontic failure. The use of fiber-reinforced composites for periodontal splinting creates an esthetic challenge in the management of the gingival embrasure area. For the replacement due to sudden loss of an anterior tooth, the pontic can be fabricated using the patient's own tooth, an acrylic denture tooth, or a tooth made from composite resin [27–30]. The placement of the pontic slightly within the healing socket can create an esthetically emerging pontic when the socket heals. It is important that the tooth pontic be slightly longer for placement slightly within the healing socket.

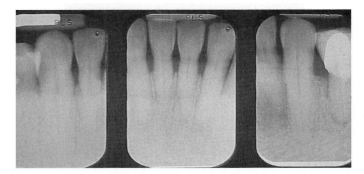

Fig. 4. Preoperative radiographs demonstrating 50% bone loss.

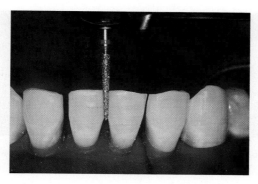

Fig. 5. The facial interproximal areas were prepared with a diamond rotary instrument.

When completing the finishing and polishing of the fiber splint, careful attention should be given to shaping the gingival embrasure interproximal areas. If there is an excess of composite resin in the gingival embrasure spaces, a Profin reciprocating handpiece with a flat Lamineer tip can be used to finish those areas. The reciprocating handpiece is used because access to the gingival margins on the proximal surfaces is limited when teeth are splinted. Finishing strips do not work well on rounded or concave root and interproximal surfaces. Likewise, the use of rotary handpieces with rotating finishing diamonds and burs often used in these interproximal areas is contraindicated because they can create unnatural embrasures and notched irregular surfaces. The reciprocating handpiece, with its back-and-forth reciprocating motion, can be used to remove excess resin and finish the gingivo-interproximal surfaces to natural form (Fig. 2). The final shaping of the gingival embrasure must permit the gingival tissues of the papilla to form a collum and adapt to the gingival areas of the tooth crown.

Case report one: mandibular periodontal fiber splint

This patient presented with the chief complaint of discomfort while functioning on the mandibular anterior teeth (Fig. 3). Radiographically, the

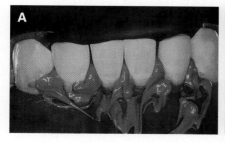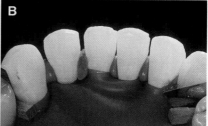

Fig. 6. The gingival embrasures with the medium-bodied polysiloxane impression materials blockout. (*A*) Facial view. (*B*) Lingual view.

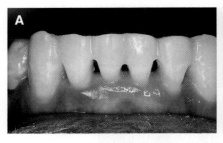
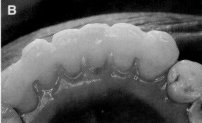

Fig. 7. Completed composite resin ribbon-reinforced splint. (*A*) Facial view. (*B*) Lingual view.

mandibular incisors had over 50% bone loss (Fig. 4) with a mobility of "2" as per the Miller's Index. The patient was referred for splinting by the treating periodontist because of secondary occlusal traumatism of the mandibular incisors. A directly placed lock-stitch, woven ribbon (THM reinforcement ribbon; Ribbond, Seattle, WA), reinforced composite resin–bonded splint extending from canine to canine was placed. For Class 1 and Class 2 occlusal schemes, the ribbon should be placed on the lingual for mandibular splints and the facial surface for maxillary splints. In the mandibular arch, the lingual approach for placement of the fiber ribbon usually does not interfere with achieving an esthetic result. For this case, a lingual splint was placed. The technique for placing a fiber-reinforced periodontal splint included placement of the dental dam, cleaning of the teeth, and minimizing bulk on the esthetic facial surface interproximally. A thin, round-end, chamfer diamond was used to prepare the facial interproximal areas (Fig. 5). The length of reinforcement ribbon was determined by placing a piece of dental floss on the facial surfaces of the incisors from the distal of the left lateral incisor to the distal of the right lateral incisor. The floss was cut to this length and used to measure and cut an equal length of a 3-mm-wide Ribbond THM ribbon, which was then wetted with bonding

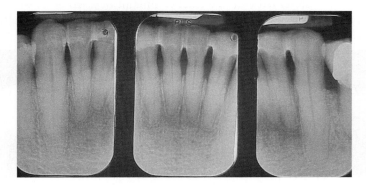

Fig. 8. Radiograph of completed splint demonstrates the x-ray–visible woven ribbon embedded in the hybrid composite resin.

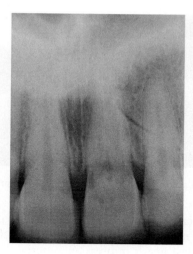

Fig. 9. Radiographic evidence of resorptive lesion on maxillary central incisor.

resin. The teeth to be splinted (#22–27) were etched with phosphoric acid on the lingual and facial surfaces that were prepared, then rinsed and dried. The most distal tooth surfaces of #22 and #27 had interproximal matrix strips placed to maintain separation. In the past, wedges were placed to minimize excess composite in the gingival interproximal embrasure areas. With wedges there is the potential that highly mobile teeth could be splinted in a different position. To minimize excessive composite resin in these areas, a medium-viscosity polysiloxane impression material was placed using an impression syringe in these gingival embrasure areas. It is important that

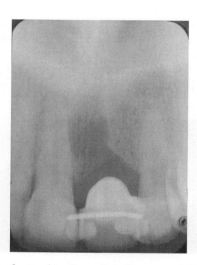

Fig. 10. Radiograph of natural tooth pontic bridge supported by orthodontic wire.

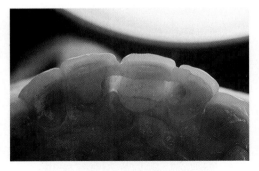

Fig. 11. Lingual preparation of abutment teeth and natural tooth pontic.

the impression material be placed after tooth etching, rinsing, and drying to avoid the trapping of moisture that can occur if the technique is done earlier (Fig. 6). This use of elastomeric impression material assures a passive placement of the blockout. A resin adhesive was painted onto the etched enamel surfaces, including the interproximal surfaces and facial interproximal areas, using a disposable brush. The resin was not light cured at this time.

A medium-viscosity hybrid composite resin was dispensed onto the facial surfaces of all the interproximal areas of the teeth to be splinted from a pre-dose tube. The facial surfaces were shaped and light-cured. The purpose of the facial composite resin was to seal the interproximal areas against recurrent caries, to provide for a 180° wrap of composite resin to each of the splinted teeth, and to stabilize the teeth to prevent movement when the composite resin and ribbon are placed onto the lingual surface. This facial extension of composite resin functions as a cross-splint for each tooth to prevent tooth movement and breakage of the final splint. Composite resin was placed onto the lingual surface, and the fiber ribbon was embedded in the composite and adapted to the teeth. Excess resin was removed, and the splint was light cured on the lingual surface tooth by tooth.

The completed splint provided tooth stabilization, increased function without bulk, and fulfilled the patient's esthetic needs (Fig. 7). The

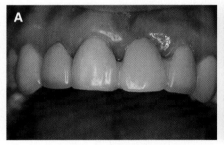
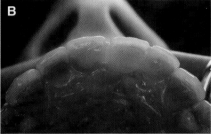

Fig. 12. Completed Ribbond natural tooth pontic bridge. (*A*) Facial view. (*B*) Lingual view.

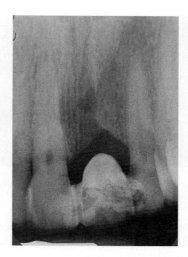

Fig. 13. Radiograph of completed bridge.

radiographs of the completed splint verify the joining of the periodontally involved incisors (Fig. 8).

Case report two: natural tooth pontic fiber–reinforced fixed partial denture

A patient who had a previous history of anterior porcelain veneers placed 2 years previously returned for a routine recall appointment, and it was noted that there was a reddish discoloration underlying the enamel of the lingual surface of tooth #9. The area was probed, and a defect on the root surface was discovered. The reddish appearance of the enamel was due to the gingival tissue that had proliferated into the root defect. A radiograph was made that demonstrated a large radiolucency at the cervical area of tooth #9 (Fig. 9). A preliminary diagnosis of external root resorption was made. The patient was referred to a periodontist and to an endodontist to evaluate the tooth's prognosis. It was determined that the tooth's prognosis was hopeless and that the tooth needed to be extracted.

The patient was presented with several alternatives to restore the site after extraction of the central incisor that included different types of fixed partial dentures, a removable partial denture, and a single tooth implant. Due to costs and other personal reasons, the patient decided to defer a single tooth implant and decided to have a natural tooth, pontic, fixed partial denture. The plan for the fixed partial denture was to fabricate it using the natural tooth crown after extraction as the pontic and joining it to the adjacent teeth with an adhesive composite resin technique using a square orthodontic wire to reinforce and retain the tooth crown.

The maxillary central incisor was removed in two stages. To preserve the porcelain veneer and tooth crown, an atraumatic method was used to

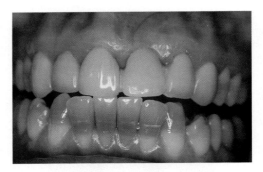

Fig. 14. Recall of Ribbond natural tooth pontic fixed partial denture at 8.5 years. (Cerinate porcelain veneers at 15.5 years).

separate the tooth crown from the root using a high-speed handpiece with a thin diamond (8392-016; Brasseler USA, Savannah, GA). The crown at the cervical line was cut slightly subgingival. Additional length for the tooth crown allows for placement of the pontic slightly within the healing socket to create an esthetic emerging pontic when the socket heals. After the incisor crown was removed, a surgical flap was used to remove the remaining root. A suture was placed to reposition the flap. The tooth crown was reshaped to be used as an ovate pontic with an adhesive composite resin restoring the root defect on the gingival surface. The natural tooth crown was joined to the adjacent teeth using a square orthodontic wire and an adhesive composite resin technique (Fig. 10).

Over the next 4 years, the fixed partial denture was repaired once, and when the patient returned with the tooth pontic loose on the distal surface due to a second fracture, the decision was made to replace the wire with a fiber reinforcement ribbon (Ribbond Reinforcement Ribbon; Ribbond). The natural tooth pontic was stabilized with adhesive composite resin on the facial interproximal surfaces in the connector region. A lingual channel 3 mm wide and equal to the width of the reinforcement ribbon was placed into the pontic, and the adjacent Class 3 composite resin was removed (Fig. 11). The length of ribbon needed was measured and cut. The fiber ribbon was placed as previously described. The fiber was embedded into the composite resin before light curing. The Ribbond-reinforced natural tooth pontic provided the patient with a highly esthetic result (Fig. 12). The postoperative radiograph shows the ribbon embedded in the composite resin (Fig. 13). At the 8.5-year recall, the fiber-reinforced fixed partial denture was highly successful. The porcelain veneers have been in placed for 15.5 years (Fig. 14).

Summary

The primary reasons for splinting and stabilizing teeth are to connect them for the purpose of replacing missing teeth or as an adjunct to periodontal therapy. Although the restorations must be planned to withstand the functional requirements of occlusion and mastication, esthetic considerations must also be taken into account. The challenge in creating an esthetic result with fiber-reinforced composite splints is that there is limited space in the connector region to create the three-dimensional effect required to give teeth the appearance of individuality. Careful planning in the diagnosis and treatment of the fiber splint is essential to allow for adequate tooth preparation to give the illusion of nonsplinted teeth. When missing teeth are replaced with a fiber-reinforced, direct, fixed partial denture, the pontic must be created to achieve an esthetically pleasing result.

References

[1] Rudo DN, Karbhari VM. Physical behaviors of fiber reinforcement as applied to tooth stabilization. Dent Clin North Am 1999;43(1):7–35.
[2] Xu HHK, Schumacher GE, Eichmiller FC, et al. Continuous-fiber preform reinforcement of dental resin composite restorations. Dent Mater 2003;19:523–30.
[3] Kangasniemi I, Vallittu P, Meiers J, et al. Consensus statement on fiber-reinforced polymers: current status, future directions, and how they can be used to enhance dental care. Int J Prosthodont 2003;16:209.
[4] Strassler HE, Brown C. Periodontal splinting with a thin-high-modulus polyethylene ribbon. Compend Contin Educ Dent 2001;22:696–704.
[5] Hornbrook DS, Hastings JH. Use of bondable reinforcement fiber for post and core build-up in an endodontically treated tooth: maximizing strength and aesthetics. Pract Periodontics Aesthet Dent 1995;7(5):33–42.
[6] Belli S, Erdemir A, Ozopur M, et al. The effect of fibre insertion on the fracture resistance of root filled molar teeth with MOD preparation restored with composite. Int Endod J 2005; 38:73–80.
[7] Ritter AV. Periodontal splinting. J Esthet Dent 2004;16:329–30.
[8] Strassler HE, Tomona N, Spitznagel J. Stabilizing periodontally compromised teeth with fiber-reinforced composite resin. Dent Today 2003;22(9):102–9.
[9] Glossary of prosthodontic terms. J Prosthet Dent 1994;71:44–111.
[10] Patzer GL. Self-esteem and physical attractiveness. J Esthet Dent 1995;7:274–7.
[11] Goldstein RE, Garber DA, Goldstein E, et al. Esthetic update: the changing esthetic dental practice. J Am Dent Assoc 1994;125:1447–56.
[12] Strassler HE, Garber DA. Anterior esthetic considerations when splinting teeth. Dent Clin North Am 1999;43(1):167–78.
[13] Pound E. Dentures and facial esthetics. Dent Surv 1962;38:35–43.
[14] Renner RP. Dental esthetics. In: Renner RP, editor. An introduction to dental anatomy and esthetics. Chicago: Quintessence Books; 1985. p. 241–73.
[15] Serio FG, Strassler HE. Periodontal and other soft tissue considerations in esthetic dentistry. J Esthet Dent 1989;1:177–87.
[16] Burger S. The arrangement of anterior and posterior teeth in the natural dentition. In: Schärer P, Rinn LA, Kopp FR, editors. Esthetic guidelines for restorative dentistry. Chicago: Quintessence Books; 1982. p. 45–69.
[17] Goldstein RE. Facial proportions: imperfect may be better. In: Goldstein RE, editor. Change your smile. Chicago: Quintessence Publishing; 1997. p. 7–8.
[18] Goldstein RE. Facing it. In: Goldstein RE, editor. Change your smile. Chicago: Quintessence Publishing; 1997. p. 1–36.
[19] Syme SE, Fried JL. Maintaining the oral health of splinted teeth. Dent Clin North Am 1999; 43(1):179–96.

[20] Hashimoto M, Ohno H, Kaga M, et al. In vivo degradation of resin-dentin bonds in humans over 1 to 3 years. J Dent Res 2000;79:1385–91.

[21] Goldstein RE. Fixed replacement of missing teeth. In: Goldstein RE, editor. Esthetics in dentistry. Philadelphia: JB Lippincott; 1976. p. 88–109.

[22] Christensen G. Fixed replacement of missing teeth. CRA Newsletter 1997;21:1–3.

[23] Vitsentzos SE, Koidis PT. Facial approach to stabilization of mobile maxillary anterior teeth with steep vertical and occlusal trauma. J Prosthet Dent 1997;77:550–2.

[24] Iniguez I, Strassler HE. Polyethylene ribbon and fixed orthodontic retention and porcelain veneers: solving an esthetic dilemma. J Esthet Dent 1998;10:52–9.

[25] Garber D, Rosenberg E. The edentulous ridge in fixed prosthodontics. Compend Contin Educ Dent 1981;2:212–23.

[26] Serio FG, Strassler HE. Perio-aesthetic troubleshooting: solutions for the unexpected. J Esthet Dent 1997;9:317–25.

[27] Ibsen RL. Fixed prosthetics with a natural crown pontic using an adhesive composite. J South Calif Dent Assoc 1973;41:100–2.

[28] Jordan RE, Suzuki M, Sills PS, et al. Temporary fixed partial dentures fabricated by means of a acid-etch resin technique: a report of 86 cases followed up to 3 years. J Am Dent Assoc 1978;96:994–1101.

[29] Strassler HE, Serio CL. Single-visit natural tooth pontic fixed partial denture with fiber reinforcement ribbon. Compend Contin Educ Dent 2004;25:224–30.

[30] Miller TE, Barrick JA. Pediatric trauma and polyethylene reinforced composite fixed partial denture replacements: a new method. J Can Dent Assoc 1993;59:252–9.

THE DENTAL
CLINICS
OF NORTH AMERICA

Dent Clin N Am 51 (2007) 525–545

Laser Use for Esthetic Soft Tissue Modification

Kenneth S. Magid, DDS[a],*,
Robert A. Strauss, DDS, MD[b]

[a]*Department of Cariology and Comprehensive Care, New York University College of Dentistry, 345 East 24th Street, New York, NY 10010, USA*
[b]*Division of Oral and Maxillofacial Surgery, Department of Surgery, Virginia Commonwealth University Medical Center, P.O. Box 980566, Richmond, VA 23298, USA*

In endeavoring to improve a patient's smile, various means of altering tooth morphology, position, and color have been used. These include orthodontics, bleaching, bonding, full porcelain jackets, and porcelain veneers. These techniques involve only tooth structure and do not address the equally important relationship of the soft tissues to the teeth or the relationship of the teeth and soft tissues to the patient's face. If disharmonies between these elements are not corrected, the resulting smile enhancement will not achieve the full desired effect.

Lasers for soft tissue and osseous recontouring

Of the means at our disposal for esthetic alteration of the soft tissues, the availability of lasers of different wavelengths provides us with the greatest range of options. Using lasers we can alter the mucosa and gingival tissues without causing bleeding, which provides better visualization, and recontour the osseous crest in a "flapless" procedure. Laser wounds exhibit histologic features that confer significant advantages over those created by scalpel or radiosurge. Most significantly, laser wounds have been found to contain significantly lower numbers of myofibroblasts, resulting in a minimal degree of wound contraction and scarring, and allowing for improved postoperative

Dr. Magid and Dr. Strauss receive compensation from Lumenis Inc. for lectures presented on the subject of laser dentistry.

* Corresponding author. 163 Halstead Avenue, Harrison, NY 10528.
E-mail address: drmagid@adfow.com (K.S. Magid).

function [1]. For esthetic dentistry, this is particularly important in dynamic soft tissues, such as those of the labial mucosa and frenum.

Frequently, the cause of a diastema and abnormal tissue architecture is a maxillary or mandibular frenum attached too close to the free gingival margin. This fibrous attachment of the lip to the alveolar mucosa may pull on the interdental papilla during lip movement, resulting in forces that separate the teeth, change the shape of the interdental papilla, and, in extreme cases, cause a malformation of the lip. In our esthetic evaluation, these tissues must be included in the overall planning to insure that the final result is not compromised. Fig. 1 shows an example of an extremely wide frenum that was attached so low it altered the contour of the lip to an unnatural, everted appearance. The frenum was excised with a CO_2 laser (Opus Duo; Lumenis, Santa Clara, CA) set on 6 W in continuous wave and attached to a focusing handpiece. The labial mucous membrane was then recontoured to eliminate the bulge of hyperplastic tissue by defocusing the laser beam and removing the tissue layer by layer in a vaporization procedure. The abnormal angle of the papilla between the central incisors was narrowed, and the gingival zenith was corrected using an Nd:YAG laser (Pulsemaster 6; American Dental Technologies, Corpus Christi, TX) set at 150 mj and 20 Hz with an initiated tip (Fig. 2).

Lasers also result in a sterile cut due to the destruction of all bacteria by the laser energy, even at low energy levels [2]. In addition, postsurgical bacteremia is greatly reduced with laser use, as a result of sealing of blood vessels and lymphatics, compared with other methods of incision [3].

When accomplishing surgical alteration of oral tissues using lasers, a thorough understanding of the physics involved and the differences between laser wavelengths is essential if a predictable outcome is to be expected. With all lasers, it is important that the operator has a thorough knowledge of laser safety and that all requisite safety measures are used for the protection of the patient and treating personnel.

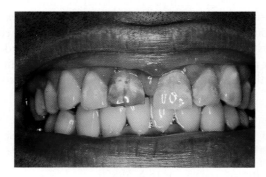

Fig. 1. Before photograph showing extremely wide and low frenum attachment resulting in the diastema between 8 and 9, everted labial mucosa, and the need for gingival recontouring.

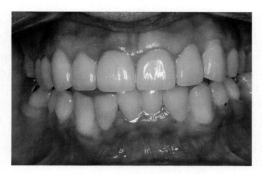

Fig. 2. After treatment with laser soft-tissue recontouring and a combination of porcelain full-coverage and labial veneers.

Laser wavelengths

Although other laser wavelengths have been used in dentistry, the following lasers are commonly used today.

Diode and neodymium:YAG lasers

Although different in their wavelengths and output, diode and neodymium:YAG (Nd:YAG) lasers are used for esthetic dentistry in a similar fashion. Both lasers penetrate deeply into soft tissue when used in a noncontact mode. When the end of the quartz fiber used to deliver the laser energy is first "activated" or "initiated" by turning on the laser and running the tip on a dark medium, such as articulating paper, the laser tip becomes carbonized. The energy of the laser beam is then absorbed by the carbonized tip, vibrating the molecules in the tip. The vibrations are converted to heat energy. As the tip heats up, it emits first red, and then orange, visible light. This can be seen as the tip reaches 900°C to 1200°C [4,5]. This "hot tip" is the mechanism by which tissue is removed without causing bleeding or substantial collateral tissue damage. The diode and Nd:YAG lasers are used in a contact mode to reshape gingival tissue. Neither laser affects tooth enamel, so they can be used in direct contact with the teeth for optimum control. Because these lasers have been shown to cause little postoperative gingival recession, cosmetic gingivoplasty can be done at the same visit as veneer preparation and impression to the new free gingival margin.

Although the diode and Nd:YAG lasers are occasionally used for frenectomy, they are limited in this function. These laser wavelengths are capable of cutting the mucosal tissue of the frenum, but the fibers that make up the true attachment are too dense for "hot tip" vaporization, and, therefore, the operator typically uses the glass fiberoptic delivery tip to cut the fibers. This does not remove the reticular fibers that insert between the teeth to permit orthodontic closure and results in substantial reattachment of a low frenum.

Carbon dioxide lasers

Carbon dioxide (CO_2) lasers have several characteristics that make them ideal for intraoral soft tissue surgery, particularly where large amounts of tissue or larger areas must be modified, such as with frenectomy or removal of hyperplasic tissue. Of great significance in the decision to use the CO_2 laser is the high degree of absorption of this wavelength by oral mucosal tissues, which are 90% water. Absorption of the laser energy by intracellular water results in a photothermal effect that is manifested by cellular rupture and vaporization. During this process, heat is generated and conducted into surrounding tissues, creating a zone of lateral thermal damage that has been found to be 500 µm or less. This lateral thermal damage also results in contraction of blood vessel walls of up to 500 µm in diameter, which is responsible for the excellent hemostasis provided by this wavelength.

When a reduction in the amount of lateral thermal damage is important, such as in gingivoplasty, modifying the output of the laser may be desirable. Control of the extent of lateral thermal damage is based primarily on the speed of the laser application. One method of reducing this "time on tissue" is to "pulse" the laser, which is possible with flashlamp or optically pumped lasers, such as erbium:YAG (Er:YAG), Er,Cr:YSGG, and Nd:YAG lasers. The faster the pulse, the less time there is available for conduction into adjacent tissues. Continuous-wave CO_2 lasers cannot be optically pumped but can be superpulsed, which is a means of obtaining high power for short periods by briefly overpumping the laser tube [6]. With a decrease in the amount of lateral thermal damage comes a concomitant decrease in the hemostatic effect of the laser. The clinician must arrive at a balance based upon the size of the blood vessels in the area and the need for hemostasis compared with the need to reduce lateral thermal damage and postoperative tissue changes.

Although CO_2 laser energy is primarily absorbed by water, it is also well absorbed by hydroxyapatite, a major structural component of tooth enamel. A significant delivery of laser energy may result in temperature changes great enough to compromise the dental pulp [7]. Commonly, errant laser energy can result in etching or pitting of the enamel [8]. It is essential that the enamel be protected while using the CO_2 laser by placing a barrier between the laser energy and the tooth or by carefully aiming the laser beam.

Erbium:YAG and Er,Cr:YSGG

Er:YAG and Er,Cr:YSGG lasers are pulsed erbium lasers whose target or "chromophore" is the interstitial water in the tissues on which they are used. Although these lasers can be used for soft tissue modification, including gingivoplasty or frenectomy, cutting is much slower than with CO_2 lasers, and the amount of laser-induced collateral thermal energy is so low that little hemostasis is provided. Although they are normally used with air/water coolant spray, these lasers can be used with little or no water, which increases the hemostatic properties to some extent but far less than that achieved with the CO_2, Nd:YAG, or diode lasers. In addition, the erbium lasers are true pulsed lasers, varying from 7 to 50 pulses per second (pps). This pulsing results in a more ragged cut than continuous-wave or "hot tip" lasers, which is a significant detriment in esthetic gingivoplasty, although the higher pulse rates have ameliorated this problem to some extent.

A significant advantage of the erbium lasers is their ability to cut bone without carbonization or scarring. Fourier transformed infrared spectroscopy has shown that the chemical composition of the bone surface after Er: YAG laser ablation is much the same as that after bur drilling, suggesting that the use of Er:YAG laser ablation may be an acceptable alternative method for oral and periodontal osseous surgery [9].

Determination of gingival versus combined osseous and gingival treatment

With each patient for whom we consider treatment with lasers, we must first determine the extent of such treatment. If the cosmetic evaluation of the patient's smile indicates the need to move the incisal edges apically, the treatment often requires the gingival architecture to move apically to provide for an esthetic length-to-width relationship, depending upon other factors, such as the patient's "high lip line" and willingness to undergo the treatment. Even when the incisal edge is determined to be in an esthetic position, evaluation of the smile includes the length-to-width ratio of the incisors and the amount of gingival and mucosal tissue displayed by the patient during smiling. Often this "gummy" smile is the main concern of the patient and must be addressed as part of the esthetic evaluation and treatment. Factors such as a hypermobile lip that exposes an inordinate amount of mucosa must be considered in the evaluation and treatment of the "gummy" smile.

Once the decision has been made to raise the free gingival margin, it is necessary to determine if this requires osseous modification and, if so, by what means. It is accepted that the normal "biologic width" (the distance from the base of the periodontal pocket to the osseous crest, incorporating the connective tissue attachment and junctional epithelium) averages 2 mm. Violating the biologic width in patients whose gingiva is "thick tissue type" results in a continuous inflammatory process, and doing so in patients who have "thin tissue type" gingiva results in uncontrolled gingival recession [10]. If raising the free gingival margin to the required esthetic height results in invading the biologic width, then osseous modification is necessary. Because lasers are "end cutting" and "side safe," a laser may be used in a novel approach to osseous crown lengthening. This "flapless" osseous crown–lengthening procedure can be used to move the osseous crest apically and change the osseous morphology such that proper contours are achieved. The healing rate after Er:YAG bur drilling has been reported to be equivalent or faster than that after bur drilling [11], and the healing rate observed

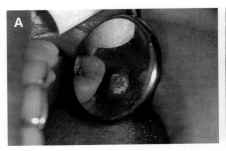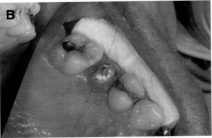

Fig. 3. (*A*) Flapless osseous crown lengthening. Osseous contours are reshaped interproximally and carried facially and lingually to achieve a periodontally stable architecture. (*B*) After 2 weeks, excellent healing and contours at the new gingival height are established.

after "flapless" crown lengthening is equally fast, usually with no evidence of the surgery after 2 weeks (Fig. 3A, B).

Procedure for flapless osseous crown lengthening

The following steps are used for flapless osseous crown lengthening:

1. Raise the gingival height and contours to the desired level using the laser wavelength of choice. The superpulsed CO_2 laser or the "hot tip" of the diode or Nd:YAG laser are excellent choices.
2. Raise the crest of bone approximately 3 mm beyond the new free gingival margin to reestablish the biologic width and normal pocket depth. Using the erbium laser, place the tip subgingivally along the long axis of the tooth until the remaining junctional epithelium and connective tissue attachment are encountered. Using approximately 200 mj and 20 pps, ablate the tissue until the crest of bone has been reached, insuring that there is sufficient water flow directed down the surgical pocket for adequate cooling of the tissues (Fig. 4). Although higher pulse rates can be provided by Erbium lasers, this increases the "time on tissue," which promotes lateral thermal damage.
3. Reduce the pulse rate to 10 pps to decrease heat buildup, and ablate the crestal bone to reestablish the desired architecture of the osseous crest at the new level (Fig. 5). It is essential that the reshaping of the bone be carried out to the outer cortical layer to avoid creating a trough in the bone. Because the side of the laser tip is not a cutting element, the tip can be used to push the soft tissue away and create the smooth desired shape (Fig. 6). The procedure is done with minimal visualization, so frequent pauses to evaluate the depth and shape of the contouring are required. A curette may be used once the bone is recontoured to smooth any irregularities and to insure proper architecture for optimal results.

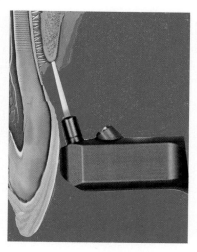

Fig. 4. Graphic showing a cross-section of the dental architecture after soft-tissue gingivoplasty and access to the crestal bone.

Although the tip is kept parallel to the long axis of the root, there is still the issue of the effect of laser energy inadvertently shining on the root surface. An experiment to determine the effect on root surfaces during calculus removal with Er:YAG laser found that root surfaces treated in vivo showed homogeneous and smooth surface morphology at settings of 120 to 160 mj [12]. When evaluated as an alternative to classic scaling and root planing,

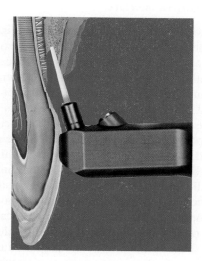

Fig. 5. The osseous crest is lowered by the erbium laser to a height necessary to reestablish biologic width at the new level.

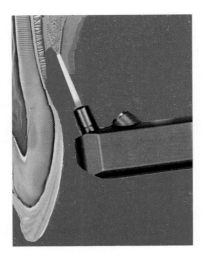

Fig. 6. Using the "safe side" of the laser tip, the soft tissues can be moved while the "end cutting" erbium laser carries the osseous recontouring out to the cortical plate.

Er:YAG lasers at 120 to 160 mj did not remove the cementum layer as would be the case with hand instrumentation [13]. In addition, Schoop and colleagues [14] found that the root surface structure of laser-irradiated roots offers better conditions for the adherence of fibroblasts than a root surface after mechanical scaling only.

Control of the tooth–gingiva interface

The visual interface of the teeth and the surrounding gingival tissues is the final element in designing soft tissue esthetics. The ideal gingival outline of the anterior sextant should be bilaterally symmetrical, with the maximal height of the gingival contours of the cuspids and central incisors on the same horizontal plane [15]. The gingival contours of the lateral incisors and bicuspids should fall slightly below this level. It is essential in anterior esthetic modifications that any discrepancy in these heights be corrected.

In correcting the position of the gingival scallop, we must also control its shape. Under normal anatomic conditions, the gingival zenith (ie, the most apical point of the clinical crown of a tooth at the gingival level) is at the junction of the middle and the distal third of the facial aspect of a tooth. This point is influenced by tooth angulation and the position of the contact point [15,16]. For optimal esthetics, the gingival scallop should not be a smooth curve but rather should peak at the gingival zenith.

The position and shape of the interdental papilla must also be taken into consideration. This is particularly important in cases where diastemas are to be closed. The interdental papilla in these areas is usually wide and blunted.

If cosmetic alteration of the teeth is done without correcting this tissue, the result will be an unnatural appearance and proximal contours that are hard to clean and do not promote gingival health.

Other modalities for tissue modification

Although this article focuses on the use of lasers in esthetics, there are other means of achieving the esthetic modifications discussed. A brief overview of the other choices in armamentarium is instructive for comparison.

Scalpel gingival recontouring

Scalpel gingival recontouring method uses small scalpel blades or periodontal surgical instruments to create the contours necessary for a pleasing esthetic result. The difficulty with this method is the resultant bleeding that obscures the operative field and the inability to use this technique at the time of preparation or impression due to the inability to achieve hemostasis. In addition, the ability of the scalpel to thin and recontour the tissues is limited. The advantage of mechanical recontouring is the lack of tissue damage beyond the cut edge and, therefore, minimal gingival recession during healing.

Apically repositioned flap

Apically repositioned flap surgery requires much more extensive surgical intervention and healing time. Because this surgery is usually beyond the scope of the restorative dentist, close cooperation and communication is required between the surgeon and the restorative dentist to insure the final result. As in scalpel gingival recontouring, it cannot be used at the time of preparation or impression but results in minimal gingival recession during healing. For most cases where altering the gingival tissues only is required, apically repositioned flap surgery is not the treatment of choice. In cases of extreme "gummy" smile where substantial osseous reduction along with gingival repositioning is the treatment of choice, apically repositioned flap surgery is a viable alternative.

Radiosurgical gingival recontouring

If recontouring of only the gingival tissues and mucosa is the desired result, a radiosurgical device can be used. The advantage of these devices is the ability to remove and reshape tissues without causing bleeding, allowing a clear view of the operative field. The difficulty using a radiosurgical device in esthetic modification is the potential for significant gingival recession after treatment due to collateral tissue damage and contracture. In

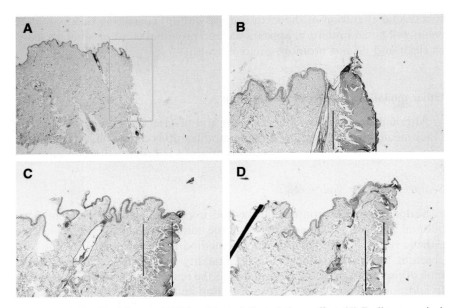

Fig. 7. (*A*) Scalpel incision on the right with no collateral tissue effect. (*B*) Radiosurgery incision using at 2.5 power intensity, fully filtered output, showing 0.5 mm of collateral tissue damage. (*C*) CO_2 incision at 8 W continuous wave with 0.3 mm of collateral tissue damage. (*Courtesy of* John Rice, PhD, Bristol, TN.) (*D*) CO_2 incision at 8 W continuous wave in superpulsed mode with 0.25 mm of collateral tissue damage.

a comparison of incisions made by scalpel, radiosurgery, and CO_2 laser, histologic evaluation shows that the scalpel incision had no collateral tissue damage, the radiosurge produced tissue damage of 0.5 mm, and the CO_2 laser had a zone of collateral thermal damage of 0.3 mm in continuous wave and 0.25 mm superpulsed wave (Fig. 7A–D). In a study that compared tissue recession after troughing (or sulcular development) before impression taking, the radiosurgery resulted in significant gingival recession in 14 out of 110 cases, whereas the Nd:YAG laser resulted in three cases of recession and the 940-nm diode laser resulted in two cases of recession [17]. If radiosurgery is used for tissue modification before veneers or other cosmetic alteration of the teeth, it is advisable to delay final preparation and impression until gingival recession has stabilized.

Case studies

Diode gingivoplasty

A patient presented with the desire to reduce her "gummy" smile, close a diastema between the central incisors, and reshape and whiten the teeth (Fig. 8). Examination showed gingival depths of greater than 3 mm, with the free gingival margin located incisal to the cemento-enamel junction,

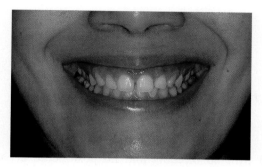

Fig. 8. Delayed passive eruption resulting in short clinical crowns and a "gummy" smile.

resulting in a diagnosis of delayed passive eruption. A discussion of gingival versus osseous recontouring resulted in the patient choosing gingival recontouring followed by porcelain veneers. During the evaluation for the gingivoplasty, the patient's anterior teeth were analyzed for angulation, gingival zenith, and the shape of the interdental papillae, especially between teeth #8 and #9 (Fig. 9).

The patient was anesthetized with one carpule of 2% lidocaine with epinephrine. An 830-nm diode laser (Diolase; Biolase, Irvine, CA) set on 3 W in continuous wave (CW) was first initiated on blue articulating paper. The laser was then used in a contact mode to resculpt the gingival tissues, reducing the periodontal pocket to no less than 1 mm. During this phase of treatment, it is essential that the practitioner keep in mind the correction of tooth position and angulation to be accomplished with the veneers so the appropriate gingival zenith and contours are established. For example, in this case, because the diastema between the central incisors was to be closed without further widening of the crown by reducing the distal enamel and adding to the mesial, effectively "moving" the crown mesially, the gingival zenith had to be moved mesially to provide an esthetic result. The angulation of the left lateral incisor would be corrected in the veneers, which would require repositioning the gingival zenith of that tooth. The gingivoplasty

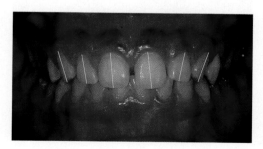

Fig. 9. Evaluation of the smile for angulation and position of the teeth indicating the necessary changes in the gingival zenith.

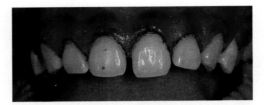

Fig. 10. After gingivoplasty using the diode laser.

was completed with no bleeding and no postoperative pain or need for medication (Fig. 10). The teeth were prepared for veneers to the new free gingival margin, impressions with vinyl polysiloxane material were taken, and the teeth were temporized. When the veneers were inserted 2 weeks later, the tissue was completely healed and the margins of the veneers were still at the free gingival margin, showing no obvious recession of the tissues after the surgery (Figs. 11 and 12).

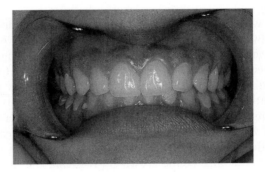

Fig. 11. Close-up of finished case with veneers. Note healing and lack of recession beyond margins. (*Courtesy of* Saiesha Mistry, DDS, and Steven Chu, DDS, MDT, New York, NY.)

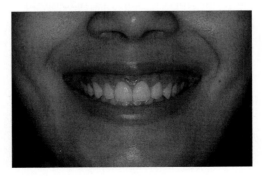

Fig. 12. Reduction of "gummy" smile, improvement of crown length/width ratio, and proper placement of gingival zenith.

Erbium:YAG osseous crown lengthening and diode gingivoplasty

A patient presented requesting an improvement in her smile. Of particular importance to this article was the discrepancy in the tissue height of the right cuspid (Fig. 13). Radiographic examination showed this to be a deciduous cuspid with a congenitally missing permanent tooth. The tooth had a substantial root structure, and the decision was made to retain the tooth rather than to perform extraction and replacement. After periodontal probing, it was decided that osseous crown lengthening would be necessary to avoid invading the biologic width. The various means of accomplishing these ends were discussed with the patient, and the decision was made to use laser osseous crown lengthening and laser gingivoplasty.

To obtain and show the excellent healing after flapless osseous surgery, it was decided to perform the crown lengthening in two distinct procedures. The first procedure was lowering the osseous crest with an Er:YAG laser (Opus 20; Lumenis, Santa Clara, CA). Because the free gingival margin was to be raised 1.5 to 2 mm, in the next procedure the osseous crest was raised to 5 mm beyond the present free gingival margin as measured by sounding the bone with a periodontal probe (Fig. 14). After 1 week of healing, which showed excellent tissue response (Fig. 15), the gingivoplasty was accomplished with an 830-nm diode laser (Diolase) set at 3 W in continuous mode with an initiated tip (Fig. 16). The veneers were prepared and temporized to the new free gingival margin. The final veneers were placed 2 weeks after surgery, with the tissue around the deciduous cuspid having healed completely and with no evidence of gingival recession. Comparing the gingival position in the initial photograph to the final position, it is easy to see the successful raising of the gingival margin to the new height (Fig. 17).

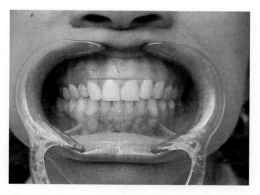

Fig. 13. Evaluation of gingival tissue showing poor height and contours of deciduous right cuspid.

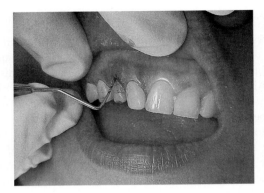

Fig. 14. Flapless osseous contouring was done, and the 5-mm height of bone required is confirmed by sounding with a periodontal probe.

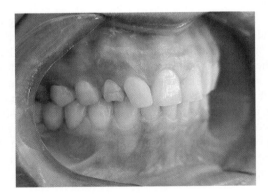

Fig. 15. One week postosseous surgery with excellent healing.

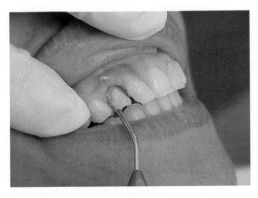

Fig. 16. Diode gingivoplasty to create desired contours.

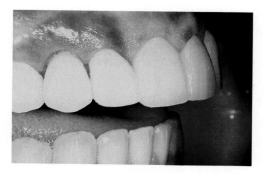

Fig. 17. Proper tissue contours achieved and veneers placed.

CO_2 gingivoplasty and erbium:YAG osseous crown lengthening

Evaluation of this patient showed a large diastema between the central incisors, malpositioning of the teeth, a high lip line, and short crown length (Fig. 18). The various options for treatment were discussed with the patient, and laser gingivoplasty and osseous crown lengthening followed by porcelain veneers was the final treatment plan.

The patient was anesthetized with 2% lidocaine with epinephrine. A CO_2 laser (Opus 20) was used at 3 W with a nonfocusing handpiece to reshape the gingival tissues. Because the energy from the CO_2 laser scars enamel, it is essential in this technique that the laser be directed at the tissue axially along the long axis of the tooth and away from the enamel (Fig. 19). The gingival zenith on the central incisors and cuspids was raised and moved mesially, as indicated by the final wax up of the veneers (Fig. 20). The shape of the interdental papilla between the central incisors was narrowed commensurately with reducing the diastema to 1 mm at the patient's request. After the CO_2 gingivoplasty, a periodontal probe was used to sound the crest of bone and determine the necessity for osseous recontouring (Fig. 21). An Er:YAG laser (Opus 20) was then used in a flapless osseous crown-lengthening procedure as described previously to reestablish the biologic width wherever it had been invaded by the gingivoplasty (Fig. 22). The periodontal probe was used repeatedly during the procedure to insure that sufficient reduction of the osseous crest had been accomplished. After surgery, all tissue

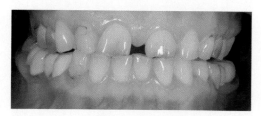

Fig. 18. Malpositioned central and gingival height discrepancies and a large diastema with wide papilla combine to create a difficult esthetic challenge.

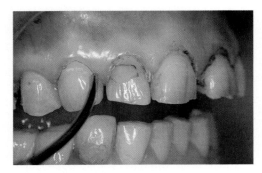

Fig. 19. CO_2 laser in a collimating handpiece aimed axially to avoid hitting the tooth as it recontours the gingival.

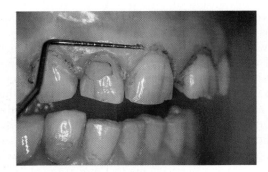

Fig. 20. Evaluation of the gingival height of #8 now higher than #7.

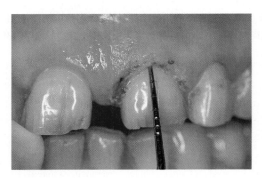

Fig. 21. Sounding the bone indicates the need for osseous recontouring.

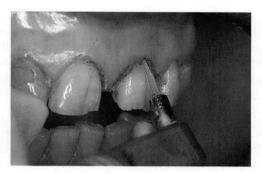

Fig. 22. Erbium laser raises the osseous crest in a flapless procedure.

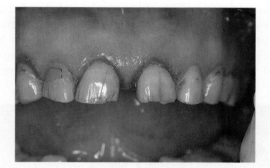

Fig. 23. All tissue contours are evaluated showing correction of gingival height and zenith and narrowing of the interdental papilla between the centrals.

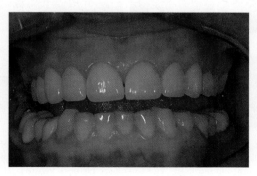

Fig. 24. Veneers in place with proper gingival contours and healing without recession (*Courtesy of* Ashish Shetty, BDS, MDS, Bangalor, India.)

contours were evaluated for gingival zenith, height, and papilla shape (Fig. 23). The patient was dismissed and examined in 2 weeks. At that time, healing was excellent, and the teeth were prepared for the porcelain veneers to the new free gingival margin. Two weeks later, the veneers were inserted with no evidence of untoward gingival recession (Fig. 24).

CO_2 correction of gingival hyperplasia

A 35-year-old man presented with hyperplastic gingival tissue secondary to cyclosporin therapy (Fig. 25A). The use of the CO_2 laser is ideal for this procedure due to its excellent hemostasis, lack of scarring, and the ability to ablate large areas by defocusing the laser. After local anesthesia, the new gingival margin was established by incising with the laser at 6 W CW in focused mode. Protection of the teeth in this technique is crucial and is achieved with a thin Freer elevator or a metal matrix band. When working in interproximal areas, an intermittent mode (50-millisecond pulses at two pulses per second) is recommended. After the excess coronal tissue was excised, the hypertrophic tissue overlying the alveolus was sculpted. This process was performed in defocused mode at 6 to 8 W using a defocused technique. This entails traversing the laser beam in a series of connecting and paralleling "U"s. This method ensures even lasing of the

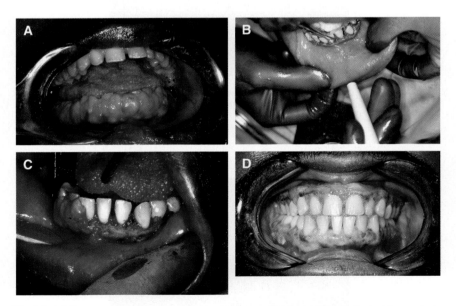

Fig. 25. (*A*) Preoperative view of a patient who has severe drug-induced gingival hyperplasia. (*B*) Using a periosteal elevator to protect the tooth from the laser beam. The red beam is from a coaxial red light aiming laser. The CO_2 laser beam is invisible. (*C*) Midway through the procedure, the hemostasis and clear surgical field are evident. (*D*) Two weeks postoperatively, the healing is excellent.

entire lesion, precluding the repetition of laser strikes at the top and bottom of the typical "V" pattern, which would double the time on tissue in those locations and increase the depth and lateral thermal damage. Once tissue has been ablated, the poor water content of the remaining carbonized surface substantially increases lateral thermal damage if lased again. Therefore, after an initial pass is performed, the surface carbonization should be gently wiped with moist gauze. If deeper ablation is desired, the next pass should be made perpendicular to the preceding one, ensuring even and complete coverage of the tissue. This ablation is continued until the desired contours are achieved [18]. After the surgery, the patient is released with no dressing or medications. The appearance of the tissues 2 weeks after the surgery is a testament to the advantages of the CO_2 laser for this procedure.

Laser punctation of perioral vascular lesions

A good cosmetic dentist realizes that esthetic results do not rest solely on the teeth or the gingival architecture. The cosmetic appearance of surrounding oral, perioral, and facial structures can have a distinct positive or negative effect on the esthetics of the anterior dentition, and the best efforts of the dentist can be enhanced or diminished by these structures.

Although alteration of facial and perioral structures is best left to a qualified oral and maxillofacial surgeon or another cosmetic facial surgeon, many cosmetic issues of the oral cavity can easily be ameliorated by the general dentist. Due to their many advantages, including the increased visibility afforded by hemostatic surgery, the use of lasers can be of great benefit in this situation. Many cosmetic issues that would be difficult to treat with other modalities are simple and safe to treat effectively with a laser.

A prime example of this is management of vascular lesions of the lips. Venous lakes, a generally harmless condition, are a common finding on physical examination of the oral cavity. Venous lakes are a collection of enlarged veins, most commonly seen in the lower lip. These nongrowing, blue, flat lesions, especially if large or multiple in nature, can be obvious and unaesthetic. An obvious vascular lesion the lip can overshadow even the most beautiful dental reconstructive effort of the anterior region.

In general, it is the goal of the laser surgeon to minimize collateral tissue damage. Lateral thermal conduction also causes vascular collagen contraction and hemostasis. Therefore, in this situation, it is desirable to maximize thermal conduction. This is accomplished by using the CO_2 laser with long pulse durations, usually in the range of 500 to 1000 milliseconds.

Fig. 26 demonstrates the use of a CO_2 laser to eradicate a typical venous lake in a 52-year-old woman. The lesions had been present for many years and had not changed in that time. When pressed upon by a clear glass slide, the lesions disappeared, confirming their vascular nature. The patient expressed dissatisfaction with the cosmetic appearance

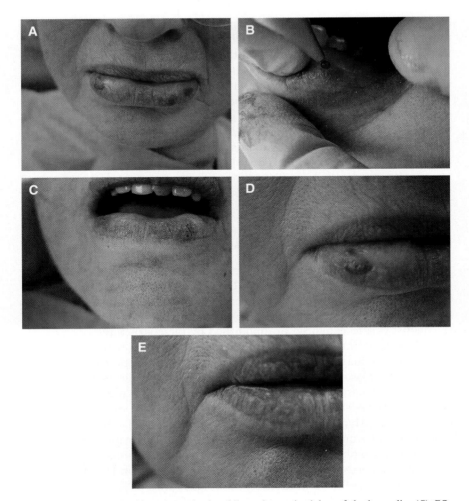

Fig. 26. (A) A 52-year-old woman who has bilateral vascular lakes of the lower lip. (B) CO_2 laser applied using 6 W, CW in 500-millisecond single pulses. (C) The lesion is eradicated with pulses placed across the lesion at 2-mm intervals. The initial bleeding is stopped after several pulses. (D) Preoperative close-up view of the right lesion. (E) Postoperative close-up view of the right lesion.

of the lesions and requested removal. After local anesthesia was administered, a CO_2 laser (Novapulse; Lumenis Inc., Santa Clara, CA) was used at 6 W CW on a setting to provide single 500-millisecond pulses. The laser pulses were distributed, one at a time, across the entire lesion at 2-mm intervals. It is not uncommon to see some bleeding associated with the initial pulses (due to the presence of any vessels with a diameter that exceeds the lateral thermal effects of the laser pulse), but this typically diminishes with each succeeding pulse. Immediate disappearance of the lesion should be seen, and any residual bleeding is easily controlled with local pressure. The patient is discharged with antibiotic ointment on the lip and with no special dietary or hygiene instructions.

Although this is a simple technique and the results are immediate and usually impressive, a proper diagnosis is critical. Lesions with a similar appearance, such as melanoma, hemangioma, or oral melanotic macule, should not be treated with this technique.

References

[1] Zeinoun T, Namor S, Dourov N, et al. Myofibroblasts in healing laser excision wounds. Lasers Surg Med 2001;28(1):74–9.
[2] Ando Y, Aoki A, Watanabe H, et al. Bactericidal effect of erbium YAG laser on periodontopatic bacteria. Lasers Surg Med 1996;19:190–200.
[3] Fisher S, Frame J. The effects of the carbon dioxide surgical laser on oral tissues. Br J Oral Maxillofac Surg 1984;22:414–25.
[4] Grant SA, Soufiane A, Shirk G, et al. Degradation-induced transmission losses in silica optical fibers. Lasers Surg Med 1997;21:65–71.
[5] Bornstein E. Method and dosimetry for thermolysis and removal of biofilm in the periodontal pocket with near infrared diode lasers: a case report. Dent Today 2005;4:62–70.
[6] Strauss RA, Fallon SD. Lasers in contemporary oral and maxillofacial surgery. Dent Clin North Am 2004;48:861–88.
[7] Powell GL, Wisensat BK, Morton TH. Carbon dioxide laser oral safety parameters for teeth. Lasers Surg Med 1990;10:389–92.
[8] Teeple E. Laser safety in anesthesia and oral maxillofacial surgery. In: Catonge G, Alling C, editors. Laser applications in oral and maxillofacial surgery. 1st edition. Philadelphia: WB Saunders; 1997. p. 46–63.
[9] Katia SM, Akira A, Ichinose S, et al. Scanning electron microscopy and fourier transformed infrared spectroscopy analysis of bone removal using Er:YAG and CO2 lasers. J Periodontol 2002;73(6):643–52.
[10] Sanavia F, Weisgold AS, Rose LF. Biologic width and its relation to periodontal biotypes. J Esthet Dent 1998;10(3):157–63.
[11] Lewandrowski KU, Lorente C, Schomacker TJ, et al. Use of the Er:YAG laser for improved plating in maxillofacial surgery: comparison of bone healing in laser and drill osteotomies. Lasers Surg Med 1996;19(1):40–5.
[12] Schwartz F, Putz N, George T, et al. Effect of an Er:YAG laser on periodontally involved surfaces: an in vivo and in vitro SEM comparison. Lasers Surg Med 2001;29:328–35.
[13] Eberhard J, Ehlers H, Falk W, et al. Efficacy of subgingival calculus removal with Er:YAG laser compared to mechanical debridement: an in situ study. J Clin Periodontol 2003;30(6): 511–8.
[14] Schoop U, Moritz W, Kluger U, et al. Changes in root surface morphology and fibroblast adherence after Er:YAG laser irradiation. Journal of Oral Laser Applications 2002;2:83–93.
[15] Sulikowski A, Yoshida A. Three-dimensional management of dental proportions: a new esthetic principle: "the frame of reference". Quintessence Dent Technol 2002;10–20.
[16] Feigenbaum N. Aspects of aesthetic smile design. Pract Periodontics Aesthet Dent 1991;3(3): 9–13.
[17] Gherlone EF, Majorana C, Grassi RF, et al. The use of 980-nm diode and 1064-nm Nd:YAG laser for gingival retraction in fixed prostheses. Journal of Oral Laser Applications 2004;4(3): 183–90.
[18] Wlodawsky RN, Strauss RA. Intraoral laser surgery. Oral Maxillofac Surg Clin North Am 2004;16:149–63.

ELSEVIER
SAUNDERS

Dent Clin N Am 51 (2007) 547–563

THE DENTAL
CLINICS
OF NORTH AMERICA

Advanced Concepts in Implant Dentistry: Creating the "Aesthetic Site Foundation"

Nicolas Elian, DDS, Brian Ehrlich, DDS,
Ziad N. Jalbout, DDS, Anthony J. Classi, DMD,
Sang-Choon Cho, DDS,
Angela R. Kamer, DDS, MS, PhD*,
Stuart Froum, DDS, Dennis P. Tarnow, DDS

*Ashman Department of Periodontology and Implant Dentistry, New York University College
of Dentistry, 345 East 24th Street, New York, NY 10010, USA*

The establishment of optimal and predictable aesthetics is one of the most important and challenging aspects of rehabilitation with dental implants. Aesthetic rehabilitation is important, not only because achieving the "perfect smile" is demanded by our beauty-oriented society, but also because individual impairment and disability may result from aesthetic deficiencies.

The goal of aesthetic rehabilitation is to alleviate or eliminate deficiencies and to obtain optimal aesthetics. Optimal aesthetics should be defined as the patient's perception of "visually pleasing or satisfying," and the clinician's assessment of acceptable anatomic architecture coupled with proper function of the masticatory system (mastication, speech, swallowing).

Aesthetic rehabilitation has to be predictable, implying reproducibility and stability of the outcome in the short and long term. Achieving these characteristics depends on the interaction between multiple variables, namely, biologic (anatomic factors, host response), surgical (procedure, technical skills), implant (dimensions, surface characteristics, design), and prosthetic factors [1]. It is obvious that analyzing, selecting, and integrating each of these factors is challenging. Because most often aesthetic rehabilitation encompasses "the aesthetic zone" of the anterior maxilla, this article

---

* Corresponding author.
E-mail address: ark5@nyu.edu (A.R. Kamer).

0011-8532/07/$ - see front matter © 2007 Elsevier Inc. All rights reserved.
doi:10.1016/j.cden.2007.03.001
dental.theclinics.com

focuses on this area. This article discusses several anatomic, surgical, and implant criteria that have to be considered to achieve optimal and predictable aesthetics. Specifically, it introduces the concepts of "Aesthetic Site Foundation", "Aesthetic Guided Bone Regeneration", and "Implant Rectangle". It helps guide the clinician in assessing anatomic factors by using morphologic and radiographic (CT scan) landmarks. Finally, the integration of the criteria described and the underlying rational are presented through illustrations and clinical scenarios.

Background knowledge

Aesthetic deficiencies may result from numerous pathologic conditions [2]. Even after a simple atraumatic tooth extraction, the alveolar ridge may lose approximately 4 mm in the buccal dimension [3]. Moreover, with tissue borne denture usage, the alveolar ridge resorption occurs at even higher rates resulting in significant ridge deformities [4]. In the maxilla, this resorption can be vertical and horizontal with buccal and palatal components significantly compromising the potential for aesthetic rehabilitation (Fig. 1) [5].

Several methods have been used to preserve and enhance the alveolar bone in the anterior maxilla before implant placement. Some frequently used ones are orthodontic tooth eruption, socket preservation, and guided bone regeneration (GBR) [6]. Although these techniques are effective in many clinical situations, they may not be sufficient in complex cases, especially where bone loss is more severe and comprises more than one aspect of the alveolar ridge (ie, vertical, buccal, and palatal). Horizontal augmentations by GBR are predictable; however vertical ones are less assured [7]. Most horizontal bone augmentations are performed on the buccal aspect of the alveolar ridge. Often the augmentation is performed purely to provide what seems to the practitioner as enough bone to cover any potential implant thread dehiscence. However, to ensure long-term stability of the soft tissue, at least 2 mm of facial bone thickness is required buccal to the implant [8]. Therefore, when a ridge deformity is complex and/or aesthetic requirements are high, it is necessary for the practitioner to have a clear

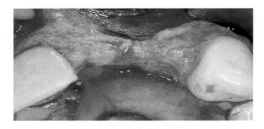

Fig. 1. Occlusal view of an anterior site showing a buccal and lingual defect. Note that the lingual defect is easily overlooked without a full reflection of the soft tissue.

vision and understanding of the three-dimensional envelop of bone surrounding an implant. Once this is achieved, the proper augmentation approach can be selected.

Another variable to be considered in aesthetic reconstruction is the bone and soft tissue remodeling following surgical intervention. The remodeling of augmented bone and the formation of the biologic width are concerns that need to be addressed. To compensate for bone resorption, the authors advocate over building of the defective ridge; this is discussed in further details in the article. Additionally, the implications that arise from the formation of the biologic width have to be considered buccally, lingually, and interproximally. For a comprehensive review of the remodeling that occurs following the formation of the biologic width, the following articles are appropriate: [9–17].

Creating the Aesthetic Site Foundation

Careful planning, superior execution, and objective evaluation of the aesthetic outcome are critical phases in the establishment of the Aesthetic Site Foundation. Important principles of each of these phases are described. The authors of this article are strong proponents of the staged approach (ie, building one step at a time based on previously successful outcomes before placing an implant into a deficient ridge), particularly in complex cases such as the ones described.

Aesthetic planning

In treatment planning an aesthetic area, the clinician must consider a manifold of important elements. Most of these have been discussed in detail in the literature. They range from evaluating broad characteristics such as facial dimensions and smile line, to detailed considerations of the delicate papilla. However, when dental implants are used in the aesthetic site, the clinician must consider another critical element: the Aesthetic Site Foundation. The edentulous ridge's osseous dimensions and contour, as well as its spatial relation to the overall aesthetic zone and tooth position are what create the Aesthetic Site Foundation. To plan for the aesthetic implant site, the clinician must determine the criteria composing the Aesthetic Site Foundation.

Criteria for the Aesthetic Site Foundation

Determination of site requirements is initially similar to all types of aesthetic evaluations. It starts with the diagnostic wax-up, necessary radiographs, mounted study models, and clinical photographs. Incisal and buccal clinical photographic views should be taken. In addition, it is important to create a radiographic template. This template should delineate radiographically the contours of the wax-up, especially the buccal and lingual location of the ideal cemento–enamel junction (Fig. 2). This template is worn by the patient during the administration of the CT scan. Evaluation of the CT scan with the radiographic template allows the analysis of the condition of the Aesthetic Site Foundation. One of the significant findings during this phase of investigation is the determination of the ridge defect spatially. It has become common to see discussion of ridge augmentations as they pertain to buccal or crestal defects. However, it is the authors' contention that therapy of the insufficient ridge cannot be approached based on buccal and crestal defects alone. In developing the Aesthetic Site Foundation, it is paramount that one also examines the following questions: does a palatal defect exist; how does the existing ridge deficiency relate to other existing structures and proposed implant position(s)? This information in

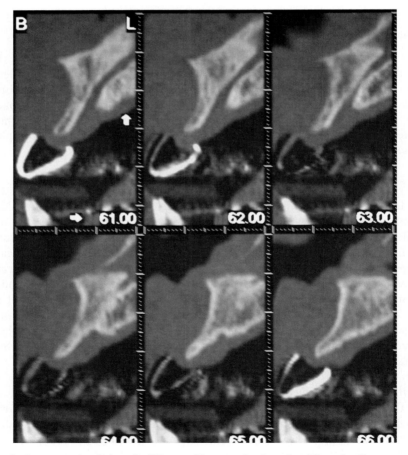

Fig. 2. A cross-sectional view of a CT scan with a complete buccal and lingual radiopaque outline of the wax up to the cemento-enamel junction. In this figure, it is clear that a buccal and lingual defect exist. Placement of an implant will result in a buccal and lingual dehiscence.

connection with the other diagnostic parameters provides the elements required for treatment planning.

Ridge defect

The standard ridge defect classification introduced by Seibert [18] is helpful during the clinical evaluation in assessing the type of deformity. Further evaluation of the ridge defect is necessary after a CT scan is taken. Addressing the combination of soft and hard tissue deformity in the vertical, buccal, and lingual dimension is of paramount importance in determining the surgical approach for the augmentation procedure (Figs. 2–4).

The goal of the augmentation procedure is to create enough bone around the implant to ensure maximum longevity of the implant and stability of the hard and soft tissue. To that end it is necessary to have 2 mm of bone thickness around the implant, especially at the crestal level (Fig. 5). This thickness is required to maintain the height of bone following remodeling of the biologic width [17]. Therefore, the authors submit the concept of the "Implant Rectangle," which is visualized in radiographic cross-sectional analysis. The Implant Rectangle is defined by superimposing vertical lines placed 2 mm buccal and 2 mm lingual to the proposed implant site, and by placing horizontal lines at the platform and at the apex level of the proposed implant. The horizontal line at the platform level is positioned parallel to the proposed buccal and lingua cemento–enamel junction and approximately 3 mm apical to it. The horizontal line at the apical level is positioned relative to the length of the implant desired and/or limitations of anatomic structures. These dimensions of the Implant Rectangle represent the minimum volume of bone required to obtain an aesthetic result (Fig. 6). Prosthetically, the buccal and lingual aspects of the tooth fall within the coronal extension of the vertical walls of the Implant Rectangle. This makes the location of the Implant Rectangle prosthetically driven. When a cement-retained restoration is planned, the implant is well within the Implant Rectangle, and the surgeon has a wide range of implants that can be used (Fig. 7). However, when a screw-retained restoration is selected, either additional volume of bone is needed at the apical aspect of the implant (in comparison to a cement-retained restoration), or a tapered or short implant is

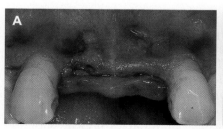 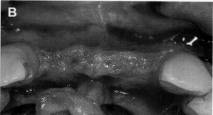

Fig. 3. (*A*) Buccal view of a deficient ridge. (*B*) Occlusal view of the same ridge.

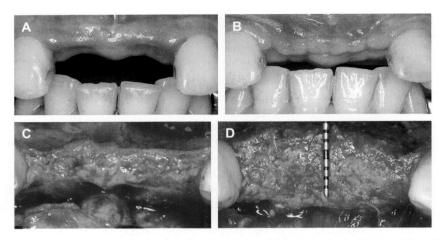

Fig. 4. Pre and postoperative Aesthetic Site Foundation. (*A*) Preoperative facial view of the soft tissue level. (*B*) Postoperative facial view of the soft tissue level. (*C*) Preoperative occlusal view of a defective ridge with buccal and lingual defects. (*D*) Postoperative occlusal view of the augmented ridge showing more than 8 mm of bucco-lingual width.

needed to keep the implant within the Implant Rectangle (Fig. 8). In summary, the *location* of the Implant Rectangle is prosthetically driven, and its *dimensions* are biologically driven. In essence, to achieve aesthetic results around implants placed in the anterior maxilla, the patient's soft and hard tissue should be transformed into a thick squared biotype. Understanding the three-dimensional criteria and the concept of the Implant Rectangle, introduced in Figs. 6–8, provides guidelines in developing the necessary augmentation for the Aesthetic Site Foundation (Figs. 9–11).

Alveolar bone of the natural tooth versus implants

In the process of developing the Aesthetic Site Foundation, the use of the CT scan delineates the deficiency found when using dental implants to replace natural teeth in the aesthetic zone. Due to the usual position of maxillary anterior teeth and the bone requirements for implants, there typically is a deficiency in the alveolar ridge for an Aesthetic Site Foundation, without surgical intervention (Fig. 12).

Limitations of the recipient site

During this information-gathering phase, factors that may hamper therapy must also be determined. These factors may include variables such as the anatomy of the surrounding area, frenums, condition of the tissue (thick or thin biotype), bone quality, medical history, medications, age of the patient, muscle pulls, and limitation of lip or cheek elasticity. For example, to what degree does the orbicularis oris muscle allow manipulation and stretching? It is imperative to fully assess all variables presented by the patient that can affect the outcome of the therapy.

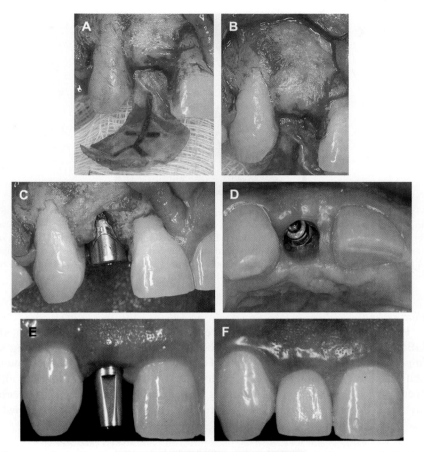

Fig. 5. Aesthetic Site Foundation: final outcome. (*A*) Re-entry view during removal of a titanium reinforced nonresorbable membrane. (*B*) Buccal view of the augmented ridge; note the overbuilding of the ridge apically. (*C*) Implant placement buccal view. (*D*) Occlusal view of the healed ridge. (*E*) Buccal view of the final abutment in place. (*F*) Buccal view of the final crown in place.

Aesthetic Guided Bone Regeneration treatment

Creating the Aesthetic Site Foundation for implant therapy involves "Aesthetic Guided Bone Regeneration" (AGBR). The protocol followed for GBR is the basic premise of AGBR. The major addition though is complementing GBR with the necessary refinements to address the issues established in the treatment-planning phase. To reach the desired level of augmentation, all aspects that facilitate surgical treatment needs to be addressed. These areas range from flap design, graft materials and membranes, scaffold design, containment, closure, postoperative treatment to secondary surgeries.

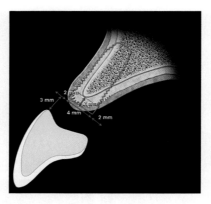

Fig. 6. In order to place an implant in proper relation to the tooth (prosthetically driven) the implant head should be approximately 3 mm apical to the buccal cemento-enamel junction of the tooth. Additionally, a 2 mm buccal and lingual bone thickness is necessary. The peak of bone facially is needed to support the soft tissue contour following the remodeling because of the biologic width. An additional 1 mm should be considered buccally and lingually for over-building during the augmentation procedure to compensate for potential resorption.

Flap design

Flap design is one of the crucial elements in AGBR. As it is with all GBR treatment, maintaining flap closure during postoperative healing is important to the success of therapy. To help in this regard, it is recommended to plan for primary closure before initiating incisions. Planning the necessary closure steps before starting surgery will undoubtedly help decide on incision lines and releasing incisions. Consideration of previously

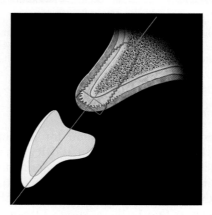

Fig. 7. Illustration of placement of an implant for a cement retained restoration. Using a 1 to 1 implant template placed on the cross section of the CT scan at the desired implant location or using planning software, the extent of the defect and the required augmentation become obvious.

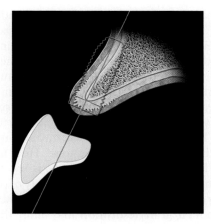

Fig. 8. Illustration of placement of an implant for a screw retained restoration. Note the required bone augmentation in comparison to Fig. 7. The apex moves buccaly, because of the lingual inclination of the head of the implant.

mentioned limitations of the recipient site should be under scrutiny. Frenums, muscle pulls, and tissue tone all need to be subjected to examination. The crestal incision is important in this regard. Often this incision is made to the palatal. However, keeping the crestal incision to the buccal will help provide for the primary closure goal already mentioned. Mesial and distal vertical releases should be placed at least one tooth away from the area to be augmented. Palatal release becomes even more critical in ridges found to be deficient on the palatal. Here proper extension of the flap will allow proper membrane and graft placement. The extent of periosteal release will vary with the degree of augmentation required as well as other anatomic factors already mentioned.

Graft materials

Numerous types of graft material have been discussed in the literature in reference to ridge augmentations. These materials can be osteoinductive or osteoconductive. They can be autogenous, allografts, xenografts, or synthetics. Their respective potential for helping form bone and the various healing times required are a topic that has been widely discussed. For the Aesthetic Site Foundation though, it is important to consider the degree of resorption that can occur with these grafts. Often, overbuilding the ridge will be beneficial in overcoming resorption. Use of a graft with less resorption is preferred.

Membranes

Membranes used in GBR can be resorbable or nonresorbable. Resorbable membranes often are made from collagen and need not be surgically removed because of their resorbable quality. Resorption varies between 8 and 24 weeks.

Nonresorbable membranes often are made from expanded polytetrafluoro-ethylene. They are also available as metal reinforced membranes (see Fig. 5). The metal reinforcement helps maintain space under the membrane. Another nonresorbable space maintainer is titanium mesh. Titanium mesh is an excellent vehicle for maintaining the desired ridge augmentation dimensions (Fig. 13). Nonresorbable membranes and titanium meshs must be removed and may create a more tenuous situation postsurgically if primary closure is lost. The selection of membrane type and/or the use of titanium mesh are important. The selection needs to take into account variables already discussed. What is the surrounding muscle tone? How much space maintenance is necessary? For example, if muscle tone is too tight, or tissues are thin, using a titanium mesh may not allow for stability of primary closure. Resorbable membranes do not create the same degree of concern should primary closure be lost, although graft resorption may limit the amount of ridge gained. The most important point about grafts and membranes is that they be properly selected based on the analysis orchestrated during the treatment-planning phase.

Scaffold

Scaffold design involves transferring the planned ridge augmentation to the recipient site. This process involves placing the radiographic template intraorally to visualize the necessary augmentation. The membrane shape and size that will provide the necessary space is then determined. The scaffold created is delineated by the membrane or mesh design used to create the necessary space. The membrane is then cut into the proper dimensions based on usual GBR membrane protocol. Allowing space for overbuilding should be kept in mind during this phase (see Figs. 9–11). One of the problems associated with current membranes are their size limitations. Often on larger defects, using a single membrane will be insufficient to create the necessary scaffold space required. It is recommended in these cases to consider using multiple membranes to create the desired AGBR ridge. In sites with buccal, crestal, and palatal defects, incorporating multiple membranes into the scaffold will be necessary to create the desired ridge augmentation (Fig. 14). Care should be taken to place the apical extent of the membrane at the required depth to allow for proper space creation. The margins of the scaffold are created by using existing heights of contour. On the ridge crest, the mesial and distal bone level is used. For the buccal, adjacent root convexity creates heights of contour mesially and distally. The palatal scaffold margins are attained by the curve of the palate or increased bone thickness on the palate. These determining factors of the scaffold margins can also act as limiting elements in creating the Aesthetic Site Foundation. These variables should be addressed during planning to help determine the expected extent of AGBR. For example, periodontal bone loss on adjacent teeth to a potential AGBR site can limit the final results. Other treatments modalities such as orthodontic forced eruption may need to be considered before AGBR.

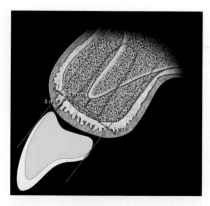

Fig. 9. Implant Rectangle. Aesthetic Guided Bone Regeneration, resulting in more than 8 mm of bone bucco-lingually, is needed to compensate for possible remolding of the augmented site. The Implant Rectangle is formed by the two vertical lines, 2 mm buccal and 2 mm, lingual to the implant and the two horizontal lines at the platform and apex of the implant. These are the minimum required volumes to obtain an aesthetic result. Note how the buccal and lingual aspects of the tooth fall within the extension of the vertical walls of the implant rectangle.

Containment

Once scaffold design has been completed, the scaffold must be secured to the ridge. A properly secured scaffold will allow containment of the bone graft. The scaffold is secured to the ridge with bone tacks, screws, or sutures. Bone tacks, placed apically on the buccal, are often sufficient for initial stabilization of the membrane. Graft material can then be added to the site. Additional tacks on the palate can be helpful with multiple membranes, or palatal defects, as long as their use does not limit scaffold spacing. Sutures can also be used to provide membrane stabilization. A horizontal periosteal suture placed at the apical area of the buccal flap extending to

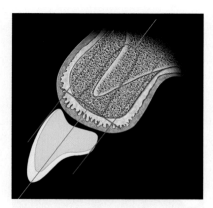

Fig. 10. Implant Rectangle. Illustration of an implant for a cemented retained restoration. Note how the implant is located well within the Implant Rectangle.

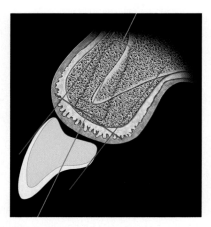

Fig. 11. Implant Rectangle. Illustration of an implant for a screw retained restoration. Note that the implant apex is close to the buccal aspect of the Implant Rectangle. A tapered or short implant may be useful to avoid a fenestration.

the palatal flap is useful in stabilizing buccal and palatal membranes over a grafted ridge. Multiple sutures done in this manner can secure the scaffold in all directions. Sutures will adapt the membrane well to all margins, making the scaffold "WaterTight" (see Fig. 14). WaterTight, is a term used to describe the relative well-contained graft within the created scaffold. Only resorbable sutures should be used in containment because they will be buried during flap closure.

Closure

Primary closure is a concern for GBR. Attaining primary closure, as described earlier, is planned during flap design. A necessity of maintaining primary closure is a relaxed flap. To attain this, a periosteal-releasing incision is

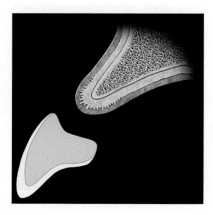

Fig. 12. Illustration of a typical defect with buccal and lingual ridge defect (as seen in Fig. 2).

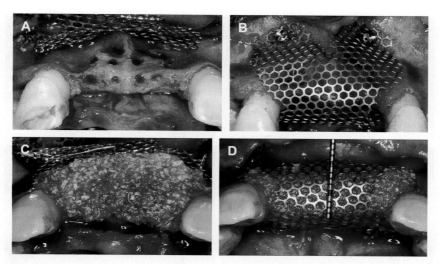

Fig. 13. Creating the Aesthetic Site Foundation. (*A*) A titanium mesh is secured in place and the recipient site is prepared to receive the graft material. (*B*) The mesh creates the scaffold for the AGBR. (*C*) Bone graft material is placed. (*D*) The titanium mesh is secured on the lingual aspect of the ridge and the site is ready for containment.

required. This incision through the buccal periosteum allows the buccal flap to move coronally. In addition, other flap manipulations are often necessary. These may include: relieving frenum pulls, sculpting or thinning tissue to allow adaptation around teeth, and pedicle or free connective tissue grafts. Resorbable or nonresorbable sutures may be used for final suturing of the flap. Initial stabilization of the buccal flap should be done with horizontal mattress sutures. Next, the mesial and distal aspects of the flap should be positioned and secured. The remaining sutures for flap margin stabilization can then be placed.

Postoperative instructions

These are the same as in a GBR procedure. The authors recommend a continuation of the antibiotic used for the surgical premedication for a minimum of 1 week. Chlorhexidine rinse twice a day for the first 2 weeks, and the patient is told not to wear any tissue borne prosthesis in the area for a minimum of 1 month, possibly longer, depending on healing. Tooth borne provisionals should be relieved at least 3 mm away from the tissue, to allow for postoperative swelling. Suture removal is usually performed during the second or third week of healing, allowing for stronger flap adhesion and for the swelling to abate.

Evaluation of the Aesthetic Site Foundation

The evaluation of the Aesthetic Site Foundation should be performed after sufficient healing time has passed. Depending on the graft used, healing

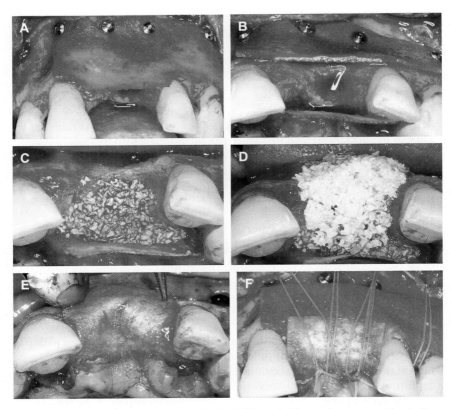

Fig. 14. Creating the Aesthetic Site Foundation. (*A*) Resorbable membranes secured apically to create the scaffold. (*B*) Occlusal view showing buccal and lingual membranes in place. (*C*) Lingual defect filled with bone graft material. (*D*) Buccal defect filled with bone graft material. (*E*) Beginning of containment: buccal and lingual membranes are wrapped over the crest. (*F*) Multiple periosteal sutures securing the membranes in place creating what is referred to as a "watertight" containment.

time can vary between 6 and 9 months. At this time the necessity for secondary procedures should be established. The detailed description of these procedures is outside the scope of this article. These procedures may include additional bone augmentations when bone foundation is still deficient and/or soft tissue manipulations. During AGBR surgery, the buccal flap is coronally advanced to achieve closure. This manipulation causes the mucogingival junction to be coronally positioned. Secondary surgery provides for correcting this displacement. During the secondary procedure, titanium mesh, nonresorbable membranes, surgical tacks, or screws should be removed. If additional soft tissue augmentation is required, it is advantageous to perform it at this time. During this phase, assessing the success of the Aesthetic Site Foundation is advisable. Postoperative CT scans taken before hardware removal, with the patient wearing the same preoperative template,

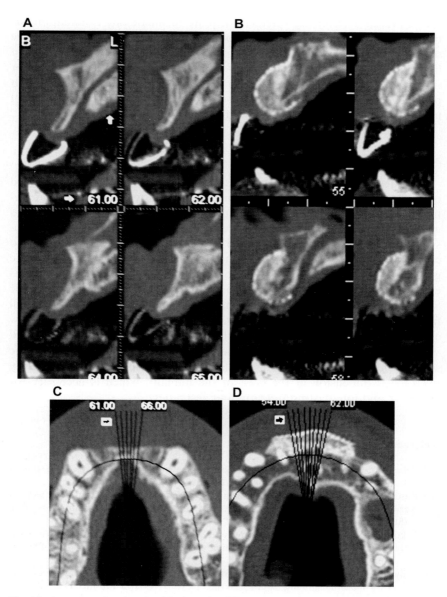

Fig. 15. A cross-sectional and axial view of a CT scan pre and post creation of the Aesthetic Site Foundation. (*A*) Preoperative cross-sectional view showing a palatal and lingual defect. (*B*) Postoperative cross-sectional view showing the creation of the Aesthetic Site Foundation. (*C*) Preoperative axial view showing a flat deficient premaxilla. (*D*) Postoperative axial view showing the overbuilt ridge.

are helpful in determining whether adequate Aesthetic Site Foundation has been created (Fig. 15). Using data from the preoperative and postoperative scans, a volumetric analysis can be performed to calculate the volume of bone that was regenerated (see Fig. 15). When the criteria necessary for the Aesthetic Site Foundation have satisfied the original goals, implant placement may proceed during the secondary surgery. Using the surgical template, the implants may be placed in the most advantageous position.

Summary

The determinants of a successful aesthetic case are interconnected and mutually dependent. The final outcome relies on careful diagnosis and meticulous execution of the planning, surgical, and prosthetic phases. In this article, the authors outlined the different criteria to consider during diagnosis and discussed the details required throughout the surgical approach to create the Aesthetic Site Foundation. Establishing appropriate diagnostic guidelines is imperative to creating outstanding successful results. To this end, the authors believe that incorporating the concept of the Aesthetic Site Foundation, the Implant Rectangle, and using AGBR techniques will facilitate producing the desired aesthetic goal-oriented results. These new concepts contrast with previously published work in terms of the required volume of bone to achieve a predictable and long-lasting result at the soft and hard tissue levels. The Implant Rectangle illustrates a frequently overlooked dimension at the crest of the implant, which is necessary for optimum and long-lasting function and aesthetics.

References

[1] Belser UC, Buser D, Hess D, et al. Aesthetic implant restorations in partially edentulous patients—a critical appraisal. Periodontol 2000 1998;17:132–50.
[2] Buser D, Martin W, Belser UC. Optimizing esthetics for implant restorations in the anterior maxilla: anatomic and surgical considerations. Int J Oral Maxillofac Implants 2004; 19(Suppl):43–61.
[3] Lekovic V, Kenney EB, Weinlaender M, et al. A bone regenerative approach to alveolar ridge maintenance following tooth extraction. Report of 10 cases. J Periodontol 1997;68: 563–70.
[4] Tallgren A. The continuing reduction of the residual alveolar ridges in complete denture wearers: a mixed-longitudinal study covering 25 years; 1972. J Prosthet Dent 2003;89: 427–35.
[5] Cawood JI, Howell RA. A classification of the edentulous jaws. Int J Oral Maxillofac Surg 1988;17(4):232–6.
[6] Salama H, Salama MA, Garber D, et al. The interproximal height of bone: a guidepost to predictable aesthetic strategies and soft tissue contours in anterior tooth replacement. Pract Periodontics Aesthet Dent 1998;10:1131–41.
[7] Esposito M, Grusovin MG, Worthington HV, et al. Interventions for replacing missing teeth: bone augmentation techniques for dental implant treatment. Cochrane Database Syst Rev 2006;25:CD003607.

[8] Spray RJ, Black GC, Morris HF, et al. The influence of bone thickness on facial marginal bone response: stage 1 placement through stage 2 uncovering. Ann Periodontol 2000;5: 119–28.

[9] Abrahamsson I, Berglundh T, Lindhe J. The mucosal barrier following abutment dis/reconnection. An experimental study in dogs. J Clin Periodontol 1997;24:568–72.

[10] Hermann JS, Cochran DL, Nummikoski PV, et al. Crestal bone changes around titanium implants. A radiographic evaluation of unloaded nonsubmerged and submerged implants in the canine mandible. J Periodontol 1997;68:1117–30.

[11] Hermann JS, Buser D, Schenk RK, et al. Biologic width around titanium implants. A physiologically formed and stable dimension over time. Clin Oral Implants Res 2000;11:1–11.

[12] Hermann JS, Buser D, Schenk RK, et al. Crestal bone changes around titanium implants. A histometric evaluation of unloaded non-submerged and submerged implants in the canine mandible. J Periodontol 2000;71:1412–24.

[13] Choquet V, Hermans M, Adriaenssens P, et al. Clinical and radiographic evaluation of the papilla level adjacent to single-tooth dental implants. A retrospective study in the maxillary anterior region. J Periodontol 2001;72:1364–71.

[14] Grunder U. Stability of the mucosal topography around single-tooth implants and adjacent teeth: 1-year results. Int J Periodontics Restorative Dent 2000;20:11–7.

[15] Elian N, Jalbout ZN, Cho SC, et al. Realities and limitations in the management of the interdental papilla between implants: three case reports. Pract Proced Aesthet Dent 2003;15: 737–44.

[16] Tarnow D, Elian N, Fletcher P, et al. Vertical distance from the crest of bone to the height of the interproximal papilla between adjacent implants. J Periodontol 2003;74:1785–8.

[17] Tarnow DP, Cho SC, Wallace SS. The effect of inter-implant distance on the height of inter-implant bone crest. J Periodontol 2000;71:546–9.

[18] Seibert JS. Reconstruction of deformed, partially edentulous ridges, using full thickness onlay grafts. Part I. Technique and wound healing. Compend Contin Educ Dent 1983;4: 437–53.

ELSEVIER
SAUNDERS

Dent Clin N Am 51 (2007) 565–571

THE DENTAL
CLINICS
OF NORTH AMERICA

Index

Note: Page numbers of article titles are in **boldface** type.

A

Abrasive compounds, natural teeth, and restorative materials, hardness values for, 386

Abrasive science, basic principles of tribiology and, 379–381

Abrasives, types and composition of, 383–384

Adhesion, dental, and dentin bonding with self-etch adhesives, 340–348
and enamel bonding with self-etch adhesives, 338–340
etch-and-rinse strategy and, 335–336
new developments in, **333–357**
self-etch strategy and, 337–352

Adhesion bridge, cantilevered, 435, 436, 437
Yamashita, 435, 436

Adhesion onlay(s), 434
metal, 434, 435
pressed ceramic bonding and, 434, 435

Adhesive joint, between enamel and etched porcelain, 333, 334

Adhesive resin cements. See *Resin cements.*

Adhesives, all-in-one, 340
clinical performance of, 349–352
etch-and-rinse, 350, 352–353

Aluminum oxide, 383

American Debtak Association, "Principles of Ethics and Code of Professional Conduct" of, 281

B

Bioactive glasses, 457

Bleaching, 313–314

Bone, and soft tissue recontouring, lasers for, 525–526

Brushes and felt devices, abrasive-impregnated, 392–393

Buccal corridor, 309–310, 312

C

Cantilevered adhesion bridge, 435, 436, 437

Carbamide peroxide, 320, 324, 327
and hydrogen peroxide, toxicology of, 322

Carbide compounds, 383–384

Carbide finishing burs, 386–387

Carbon dioxide gingivoplasty, and erbium:YAG osseous crown lengthening, 539–542

Carbon dioxide lasers, 528
for correction of gingival hyperplasia, 542–543
to eradicate venous lakes, 543–545

Cements, adhesive resin. See *Resin cements.*
commercially available, 453–454
for use in esthetic dentistry, **453–471**
glass ionomer, 456–457
luting, 400–401
material classes of, 454, 455
requirements of, 453
zinc phosphate, 454

Ceramics, nonetchable, for porcelain adhesion, 443, 446–447
"pressed," 433
bonding with, and adhesion onlays, 434, 435

Chlorhexidine, 457

Color management, predictable, in esthetic restorative dentistry, clinical steps to, **473–485**

Composite esthetic restorations, adhesives and techniques, 363
anterior, direct placement of, **359–377**

Moving?

Make sure your subscription moves with you!

To notify us of your new address, find your **Clinics Account Number** (located on your mailing label above your name), and contact customer service at:

E-mail: elspcs@elsevier.com

800-654-2452 (subscribers in the U.S. & Canada)
407-345-4000 (subscribers outside of the U.S. & Canada)

Fax number: 407-363-9661

Elsevier Periodicals Customer Service
6277 Sea Harbor Drive
Orlando, FL 32887-4800

*To ensure uninterrupted delivery of your subscription, please notify us at least 4 weeks in advance of move.